Pancreatobiliary Pathology

Editor

AATUR D. SINGHI

SURGICAL PATHOLOGY CLINICS

www.surgpath.theclinics.com

Consulting Editor
JASON L. HORNICK

September 2022 • Volume 15 • Number 3

ELSEVIER

1600 John F. Kennedy Boulevard ● Suite 1800 ● Philadelphia, Pennsylvania, 19103-2899

http://www.theclinics.com

SURGICAL PATHOLOGY CLINICS Volume 15, Number 3
September 2022 ISSN 1875-9181, ISBN-13: 978-0-323-91973-9

Editor: Taylor Hayes
Developmental Editor: Diana Grace Ang

Surgical Pathology Clinics (ISSN 1875-9181) is published quarterly by Elsevier Inc., 360 Park Avenue South, New York, NY 10010. Months of issue are March, June, September, and December. Business and Editorial Office: Elsevier Inc., 1600 John F. Kennedy Blvd., Ste. 1800, Philadelphia, PA 19103-2899. Accounting and Circulation Offices: Elsevier Inc., 3251 Riverport Lane, Maryland Heights, MO 63043. Periodicals postage paid at New York, NY and at additional mailing offices. Subscription prices are $237.00 per year (US individuals), $376.00 per year (US institutions), $100.00 per year (US students/residents), $283.00 per year (Canadian individuals), $395.00 per year (Canadian Institutions), $284.00 per year (foreign individuals), $395.00 per year (foreign institutions), and $120.00 per year (international students/residents), $100.00 per year (Canadian students/residents). Foreign air speed delivery is included in all *Clinics'* subscription prices. All prices are subject to change without notice. **POSTMASTER:** Send address changes to *Surgical Pathology Clinics*, Elsevier, 3251 Riverport Lane, Maryland Heights, MO 63043. **Customer Service: 1-800-654-2452 (US). From outside the United States, call 1-314-447-8871. Fax: 1-314-447-8029. E-mail:** JournalsCustomerServiceusa@elsevier.com **(for print support)** and JournalsOnlineSupport-usa@elsevier.com **(for online support).**

Reprints. For copies of 100 or more, of articles in this publication, please contact the Commercial Reprints Department, Elsevier Inc., 360 Park Avenue South, New York, NY 10010-1710. Tel. 212-633-3874; Fax: 212-633-3820; E-mail: reprints@elsevier.com.

Surgical Pathology Clinics of North America is covered in *MEDLINE/PubMed (Index Medicus).*

Contributors

CONSULTING EDITOR

JASON L. HORNICK, MD, PhD
Director of Surgical Pathology and
Immunohistochemistry, Brigham and Women's
Hospital, Professor of Pathology, Harvard
Medical School, Boston, Massachusetts, USA

EDITOR

AATUR D. SINGHI, MD, PhD
Department of Pathology, University of
Pittsburgh, University of Pittsburgh Medical
Center, Pittsburgh, Pennsylvania, USA

AUTHORS

HEBA ABDELAL, MD
Department of Pathology, Yale School of
Medicine, New Haven, Connecticut, USA

DANIELA S. ALLENDE, MD, MBA
Robert J. Tomsich Pathology & Laboratory
Medicine Institute, Cleveland Clinic, Cleveland,
Ohio, USA

HUSSEIN A. ASSI, MD
Department of Medicine, Boston University
School of Medicine, Boston, Massachusetts,
USA

AHMED BAKHSHWIN, MD
Robert J. Tomsich Pathology & Laboratory
Medicine Institute, Cleveland Clinic, Cleveland,
Ohio, USA

PHOENIX D. BELL, MD, MS
Department of Pathology, University of
Pittsburgh Medical Center, Pittsburgh,
Pennsylvania, USA

MELENA D. BELLIN, MD, MS
Professor, Department of Pediatrics and
Department of Surgery, University of
Minnesota Medical School, Minneapolis,
Minnesota, USA

EMILY R. BRAMEL
PhD Student, Division of Liver Diseases,
Department of Medicine, Tisch Cancer
Institute, Icahn School of Medicine at
Mount Sinai, New York, New York,
USA

LODEWIJK A.A. BROSENS, MD, PhD
Department of Pathology, University Medical
Center Utrecht, Utrecht University, Utrecht, the
Netherlands

DEYALI CHATTERJEE, MD
Department of Pathology, The University of
Texas MD Anderson Cancer Center, Houston,
Texas, USA

ANA DE JESUS-ACOSTA, MD
Department of Oncology, The Sidney
Kimmel Comprehensive Cancer Center at
Johns Hopkins, Johns Hopkins School of
Medicine, Baltimore, Maryland,
USA

SADÉ M.B. FINN, MD
Department of Surgery, University of
Minnesota Medical School, Minneapolis,
Minnesota, USA

WENZEL M. HACKENG, MD, PhD
Department of Pathology, University Medical Center Utrecht, Utrecht University, Utrecht, the Netherlands

CHRISTOPHER M. HEAPHY, PhD
Departments of Medicine, and Pathology and Laboratory Medicine, Boston University School of Medicine, Boston, Massachusetts, USA

CAROLINE F. HILBURN, MD
Department of Pathology, Massachusetts General Hospital, Boston, Massachusetts, USA

NESTEENE JOY PARAM
PhD Student, Department of Oncological Sciences, Tisch Cancer Institute, Icahn School of Medicine at Mount Sinai, New York, New York, USA

CLAUDIO LUCHINI, MD, PhD
Department of Diagnostics and Public Health, Section of Pathology, University and Hospital Trust of Verona, Verona, Italy

ANIRBAN MAITRA, MD
Department of Translational Molecular Pathology, Sheikh Ahmed Center for Pancreatic Cancer Research, The University of Texas MD Anderson Cancer Center, Houston, Texas, USA

FLORENCIA McALLISTER, MD
Department of Clinical Cancer Prevention, Clinical Cancer Genetics Program, Department of Gastrointestinal Medical Oncology, Department of Immunology, The University of Texas MD Anderson Cancer Center, Houston, Texas, USA

CHIRAYU MOHINDROO, MD
Department of Clinical Cancer Prevention, The University of Texas MD Anderson Cancer Center, Houston, Texas, USA; Department of Internal Medicine, Sinai Hospital of Baltimore, Baltimore, Maryland, USA

MAUREEN MORK, MS
Clinical Cancer Genetics Program, The University of Texas MD Anderson Cancer Center, Houston, Texas, USA

ALESSANDRO PANICCIA, MD
Assistant Professor of Surgery, Division of Surgical Oncology, University of Pittsburgh Medical Center, Pittsburgh, Pennsylvania, USA

MARTHA B. PITMAN, MD
Professor of Pathology, Harvard Medical School, Director of Cytopathology, Massachusetts General Hospital, Boston, Massachusetts, USA

DANIELA SIA, PhD
Assistant Professor, Division of Liver Diseases, Liver Cancer Program, Department of Medicine, Tisch Cancer Institute, Icahn School of Medicine at Mount Sinai, New York, New York, USA

AATUR D. SINGHI, MD, PhD
Department of Pathology, University of Pittsburgh, University of Pittsburgh Medical Center, Pittsburgh, Pennsylvania, USA

ELIZABETH D. THOMPSON, MD, PhD
Department of Pathology, Department of Oncology, Johns Hopkins School of Medicine, Baltimore, Maryland, USA

VASSILENA TSVETKOVA, MD, PhD
Department of Diagnostics and Public Health, Section of Pathology, University and Hospital Trust of Verona, Verona, Italy

CHRISTOPHER J. VANDENBUSSCHE, MD, PhD
Departments of Pathology and Oncology, Johns Hopkins School of Medicine, Baltimore, Maryland, USA

FLORINE H.M. WESTERBEKE, BSc (Med)
Department of Pathology, University Medical Center Utrecht, Utrecht University, Utrecht, the Netherlands

MATTHEW B. YURGELUN, MD
Department of Medical Oncology, Dana-Farber Cancer Institute, Boston, Massachusetts, USA

M. LISA ZHANG, MD
Department of Pathology, Massachusetts General Hospital, Boston, Massachusetts, USA

JIAN ZHENG, MD
Complex General Surgical Oncology Fellow,
Division of Surgical Oncology, University of
Pittsburgh Medical Center, Pittsburgh,
Pennsylvania, USA

AMER H. ZUREIKAT, MD, FACS
Professor and Chief, Division of Surgical
Oncology, University of Pittsburgh
Medical Center, Pittsburgh, Pennsylvania,
USA

Contents

> Examination of fine needle aspirations and small core biopsies of the pancreas can
> be an extremely difficult and treacherous area for the diagnostic pathologist. The
> pancreas often yields small and often fragmented specimens, which, in combination
> with the morphologic overlap between numerous neoplastic and nonneoplastic
> mimickers, generate multiple potential diagnostic pitfalls. The authors review this
> challenging topic and provide insight into resolving these pitfalls using morphologic
> pattern recognition and ancillary testing.

> Pancreatic cystic lesions are found in approximately 2% of the general population.
> Up to 15% of mucinous pancreatic cystic lesions (which include mucinous cystic
> neoplasms and intraductal papillary mucinous neoplasms) give rise to pancreatic
> ductal adenocarcinoma. Due to their premalignant nature, it is important to detect
> mucinous cysts early for optimal managmement. Recently, molecular analysis of
> pancreatic cyst fluid has been able to stratify patients with PCLs into those with
> low or high-risk of progression.

> Biliary duct brushing cytology is the standard of care for the assessment of bile duct
> strictures but suffers from low sensitivity for the detection of a high-risk stricture.
> Pathologic diagnosis of strictures is optimized by integration of cytomorphology
> and molecular analysis with fluorescence in situ hybridization or next-generation
> sequencing. Bile duct cancers are genetically heterogeneous, requiring analysis of
> multiple gene panels to increase sensitivity. Using molecular analysis as an ancillary
> test for bile duct brushing samples aids in the identification of mutations that support
> the diagnosis of a high-risk stricture as well as the identification of actionable muta-
> tions for targeted therapies currently in clinical trials for the treatment of patients with
> bile duct cancer.

> Three recent advances in the surgical approach to pancreatic cancer over the past
> decade have improved both short- and long-term outcomes for patients with non-
> metastatic, operable pancreatic cancer. These include (1) minimally invasive
> pancreatectomy to reduce operative morbidity while adhering to principles of
> open oncologic resections, (2) neoadjuvant chemotherapy to treat radiographically

occult metastatic disease and improve locoregional control, and (3) applying irreversible electroporation as an adjunct to surgery, allowing a fraction of locally advanced pancreatic cancer to be resected.

Identification of deleterious germline mutations in pancreatic ductal adenocarcinoma (PDAC) patients can have therapeutic implications for the patients and result in cascade testing and prevention in their relatives. Universal testing for germline mutations is now considered standard of care in patients with PDAC, regardless of family history, personal history, or age. Here, we highlight the commonly identified germline mutations in PDAC patients as well as the impact of multigene panel testing. We further discuss therapeutic implications of germline testing on the index cases, and the impact of cascade testing on cancer early detection and prevention in relatives.

Total pancreatectomy with islet autotransplantation (TPIAT) is a surgical procedure undertaken in some patients with severe pain or disability from recurrent acute and chronic pancreatitis (CP). TPIAT provides a rare opportunity to study human pancreas tissue from patients affected with pancreatitis, and particularly from patients with genetic forms of pancreatitis. Research to date suggests distinct histopathology and potentially differential pathophysiology of distinct etiologies of CP. Histopathology specimens have helped better define the success and limitations of clinical diagnostic imaging tools, such as magnetic retrograde cholangiopancreatography and endoscopic ultrasound.

Examination of pancreatic ductal adenocarcinoma after NAT with the intent of diagnosis and outcome prediction remains a challenging task. The lack of a uniform approach to macroscopically assess these cases along with variations in sampling adds to the complexity. Several TRG systems have been proposed to correlate with an overall survival. In clinical practice, most of these TRG schemes have shown low level of interobserver agreement arguing for a need of larger studies and more innovative ways to assess outcome in this population.

Cholangiocarcinoma (CCA) is a group of malignancies of the bile ducts with high mortality rates and limited treatment options. In the past decades, remarkable efforts have been dedicated toward elucidating the specific molecular signaling pathways and oncogenic loops driving cholangiocarcinogenesis to ultimately develop more effective therapies. Despite some recent advances, an extensive intra- and inter-tumor heterogeneity together with a poorly understood immunosuppressive microenvironment significantly compromises the efficacy of available treatments. Here, we provide a concise review of the latest advances and current knowledge of the molecular pathogenesis of CCA focusing on clinically relevant aberrations as well as future research avenues.

Wenzel M. Hackeng, Hussein A. Assi, Florine H.M. Westerbeke, Lodewijk A.A. Brosens, and Christopher M. Heaphy

Pancreatic neuroendocrine tumors (PanNETs) represent a clinically challenging disease because these tumors vary in clinical presentation, natural history, and prognosis. Novel prognostic biomarkers are needed to improve patient stratification and treatment options. Several putative prognostic and/or predictive biomarkers (eg, alternative lengthening of telomeres, ATRX/DAXX loss) have been independently validated. Additionally, recent transcriptomic and epigenetic studies focusing on endocrine differentiation have identified PanNET subtypes that display similarities to either α-cells or β-cells and differ in clinical outcomes. Thus, future prospective studies that incorporate genomic and epigenetic biomarkers are warranted and have translational potential for individualized therapeutic and surveillance strategies.

Vassilena Tsvetkova and Claudio Luchini

Pancreatic mixed neuroendocrine-non-neuroendocrine neoplasms (MiNENs) are rare neoplasms, composed of at least two components. The neuroendocrine part is always present. Histology is the most important tool for the diagnosis, but in the case of MiNEN, it is also important the use of immunohistochemistry, which should include neuroendocrine but also ductal and acinar markers. Each component should be specifically described in the final pathology report, including the percentage on the entire tumor mass. The prognosis of MiNEN is very heterogeneous and depends on the different tumor components.

Heba Abdelal and Deyali Chatterjee

Intracholecystic papillary-tubular neoplasm denotes a discrete mucosal-based neoplastic proliferation into the gallbladder lumen. It is diagnosed incidentally during cholecystectomy or radiologically during any workup. The majority of polypoid lesions in the gallbladder are non-neoplastic; therefore, pathologic examination is the gold standard to establish this diagnosis. Intracholecystic papillary-tubular neoplasm is considered as premalignant, although associated invasive carcinomas may be present in the specimen. Invasive carcinoma arising from intracholecystic papillary-tubular neoplasm have a better prognosis than de novo gallbladder carcinomas. The pathology of intracholecystic papillary-tubular neoplasm, including the challenges involved in the diagnosis of this entity, is discussed.

SURGICAL PATHOLOGY CLINICS

SERIES OF RELATED INTEREST

Clinics in Laboratory Medicine
http://www.labmed.theclinics.com/
Medical Clinics
https://www.medical.theclinics.com/

THE CLINICS ARE AVAILABLE ONLINE!
Access your subscription at:
www.theclinics.com

Preface

The Evolving Clinical, Pathologic, and Molecular Landscape of Pancreatobiliary Diseases

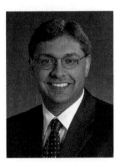

Aatur D. Singhi, MD, PhD
Editor

Pancreatobiliary diseases represent a heterogeneous and complex group of disorders that span a diverse number of benign and malignant conditions. Within the past few decades, there has been a dramatic increase in patients afflicted with these diseases. In addition, the diagnosis of many pancreatobiliary disorders has been a formidable challenge and has resulted in a significant burden on current health care resources. The treatment of pancreatobiliary diseases can also be associated with considerable patient morbidity and mortality. Despite these issues, there have been several advancements, improvements, and refinements to multiple aspects of our understanding of the pathobiology, clinical presentation, diagnosis, management, and follow-up of various pancreatobiliary disorders.

Within this issue of *Surgical Pathology Clinics*, rather than providing a broad but brief overview of pancreatobiliary diseases, we focus on important updates within the field by a diverse group of

leading experts. The first set of reviews covers a particularly difficult area, which is early detection of both pancreatic and biliary neoplasms. The authors discuss recent improvements in the preoperative evaluation of pancreatobiliary lesions to include the interpretation of small-core biopsy needles and the integration of molecular testing to pancreatobiliary specimens that can be a useful adjunct in establishing a diagnosis of not only neoplastic lesions but also nonneoplastic lesions. The next group of reviews focuses on evolving treatment strategies for pancreatobiliary cancers, such as the clinical utility and ramifications of germline testing that have become standard of care for all pancreatic cancer patients, and surgical workup and management of pancreatobiliary neoplasms. The final set of reviews represents a potpourri of information that discusses challenging areas of pancreatobiliary pathology: chronic pancreatitis from the perspective of total pancreatectomy and islet autotransplantation,

Surgical Pathology 15 (2022) xi–xii
https://doi.org/10.1016/j.path.2022.06.001
1875-9181/22/© 2022 Published by Elsevier Inc.

the histopathology of neoadjuvant-treated pancreatic ductal adenocarcinoma, the molecular pathogenesis and associated targeted therapies for cholangiocarcinoma, emerging biomarkers for pancreatic neuroendocrine tumors, and novel diagnostic entities, such as mixed neuroendocrine-nonneuroendocrine neoplasms of the pancreas and intracholecystic papillary-tubular neoplasms of the gallbladder. It is our hope that this group of in-depth reviews will be a resource for not only pathologists but also gastroenterologists, surgeons, oncologists, researchers, and, importantly, patients.

Aatur D. Singhi, MD, PhD
University of Pittsburgh
University of Pittsburgh Medical Center
Department of Pathology
200 Lothrop Street, Room A616.2
Pittsburgh, PA 15213, USA

E-mail address:
singhiad@upmc.edu

The Diagnostic Challenge of Evaluating Small Biopsies from the Pancreatobiliary System

Elizabeth D. Thompson, MD, PhD[a,b], M. Lisa Zhang, MD[c],
Christopher J. VandenBussche, MD, PhD[a,b],*

KEYWORDS

• Pancreas • Pancreatic • Fine needle aspiration • Cytology • Cytopathology • Biopsy

---

Key Points

- Loss of labeling for Smad4 (Dpc4) in atypical glands within the pancreas is highly specific for adenocarcinoma, however, intact expression is unhelpful as a portion of adenocarcinomas will show intact expression.

- Autoimmune pancreatitis can mimic adenocarcinoma, both radiographically and histologically. The classic inflammatory changes in both types, as well as elevation of IgG4+ plasma cells in Type 1, can be patchy and poorly represented on biopsy.

- Features of rare subtypes of adenocarcinoma such as adenosquamous carcinoma can be difficult to appreciate on small core biopsies but their presence should be actively sought as they have the potential to change management in the neoadjuvant setting.

- When diagnosed by FNA, well-differentiated ductal adenocarcinomas should be distinguished from benign gastrointestinal contamination and reactive atypia seen in ductal epithelium, especially in the setting of chronic pancreatitis.

- The presence of *KRAS* and *GNAS* mutations is highly sensitive for mucinous cysts (with *GNAS* being specific for intraductal papillary mucinous neoplasm) and the presence of alterations in *TP53*, *p16/CDKN2A*, *SMAD4*, *PIK3CA*, *PTEN*, and others can signal high-grade dysplasia or invasive carcinoma.

ABSTRACT

Examination of fine needle aspirations and small core biopsies of the pancreas can be an extremely difficult and treacherous area for the diagnostic pathologist. The pancreas often yields small and often fragmented specimens, which, in combination with the morphologic overlap between numerous neoplastic and nonneoplastic mimickers, generate multiple potential diagnostic pitfalls. The authors review this challenging topic and provide insight into resolving these pitfalls using morphologic pattern recognition and ancillary testing.

INTRODUCTION

Examination of fine needle aspirations and small core biopsies of the pancreas can be an extremely treacherous area for the diagnostic pathologist. The pancreas is difficult to access and typically yields small and fragmented specimens, which, in combination with morphologic overlap between numerous neoplastic and nonneoplastic

---

[a] Department of Pathology, The Johns Hopkins University School of Medicine, 600 N. Wolfe St., Baltimore, MD, USA; [b] Department of Oncology, The Johns Hopkins University School of Medicine, 600 N. Wolfe St., Baltimore, MD, USA; [c] Department of Pathology, Massachusetts General Hospital, 55 Fruit St., Boston, MA 02114 USA
* Corresponding author. The Johns Hopkins University School of Medicine, Pathology Room 406, 600 North Wolfe Street, Baltimore, MD 21287.
E-mail address: cjvand@jhmi.edu

Surgical Pathology 15 (2022) 435–453
https://doi.org/10.1016/j.path.2022.05.001

mimickers, generate multiple potential diagnostic pitfalls. Morphologic pattern recognition and ancillary testing can help overcome these pitfalls.

ADENOCARCINOMA

The intact tissue architecture present on small core biopsies of the pancreas can allow for both the diagnosis of adenocarcinoma and evaluation of invasion. However, the nature of tissue cores derived from endoscopic ultrasound-guided procedures are often thin, fragmented and hemorrhagic, generating significant challenges for pathologists. Fragmentation of cores can lead to displacement of both neoplastic and nonneoplastic epithelium into stromal tissue, mimicking invasion. The displacement of small, atrophic ducts, such those seen in chronic pancreatitis, is particularly problematic as this can create an illusion of angulation and infiltration. Careful attention should be paid to the possibility of displacement when tissue cores are particularly fragmented. The tendency toward fragmentation in pancreatic tissue cores may also lead to a biopsy where the neoplastic components are entirely detached from surrounding stroma (**Fig. 1**). In this case, high-grade dysplasia arising in a precursor lesion such as an intraductal papillary mucinous neoplasm (IPMN) cannot be distinguished from detached fragments of invasive adenocarcinoma without knowledge of the radiographic findings (solid or cystic lesion). Caution should be applied when interpreting these biopsies and careful correlation with the imaging is necessary.

Even with the benefit of architecture afforded by a core biopsy, the diagnosis of invasive adenocarcinoma can still be quite challenging. Several features can be used to favor the diagnosis of adenocarcinoma (**Box** 1). The infiltrative growth pattern of invasive adenocarcinoma contrasted with the maintenance of a lobulated architecture in chronic pancreatitis is very helpful even at low power magnification (**Fig. 2**). In more advanced parenchymal atrophy with extensive loss of acinar tissue, clues to a lobulated architecture are subtler but can still assist in preventing the pitfall of interpreting atrophic benign glands as malignant infiltrative glands (**Fig. 3**). Atrophic lobules will maintain separation from each other as well as a crisp interface with nerves and vessels found at the periphery of lobules. In contrast, when present on core biopsy, the following features can be diagnostic of invasive adenocarcinoma: infiltrative growth around muscular vessels, perineural invasion, glands present within thick smooth muscle, or within skeletal muscle (**Fig. 4**). A potential pitfall to be mindful of when evaluating the presence of glands within muscle is whether the biopsy could have traversed the ampulla, as normal ampullary glands lacking cytologic atypia will be associated with smaller, more delicate smooth muscle bundles of the sphincter of Oddi. The fibrosis associated with chronic pancreatitis can also take on a blue-gray tone usually associated with desmoplasia, and care should be taken not to overinterpret these stromal changes around benign, atrophic-appearing lobules.

In certain biopsies, infiltrative-appearing glands may lack cytologic atypia, or atypical glands may have insufficient evidence of infiltration on H&E. These cases may be very suspicious for adenocarcinoma but can lead to significant discomfort in making a definitive diagnosis on a small core. In such cases, ancillary immunohistochemistry for Smad4 (Dpc4) and p53 proteins can be helpful. *SMAD4* is a tumor suppressor showing allelic

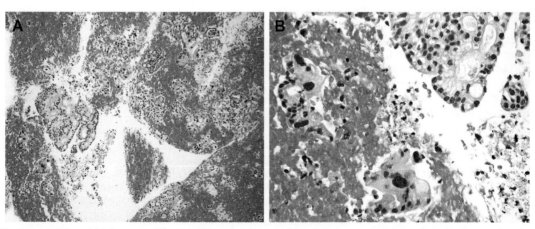

Fig. 1. Low (*A*) and high-power (*B*) magnification of a core biopsy from a pancreatic adenocarcinoma showing entirely detached neoplastic epithelium.

Box 1
Features supporting adenocarcinoma over chronic pancreatitis on core biopsy specimens

Haphazard growth pattern

Incomplete lumina/luminal necrosis

Nuclear size variation greater than 4:1

Growth next to muscular vessel

Perineural invasion

Vascular invasion

Ancillary IHC: loss of immunolabeling for Smad4

---

inactivation in about 55% to 60% of pancreatic ductal adenocarcinomas.[1] Immunohistochemistry for Smad4 protein correlates tightly with genomic status, and labeling will be lost in up to 60% of adenocarcinomas and will be universally intact in benign ducts.[2] Loss of labeling for Smad4 (Dpc4) in atypical glands within the pancreas is highly specific for adenocarcinoma (Fig. 5); however, intact expression is unhelpful as a portion of

adenocarcinomas will show intact expression. In addition, interpretation of the Smad4 immunostain can be challenging because the stain is often weak. A high threshold is recommended for interpreting the stain as lost in tumor cells (complete nuclear and cytoplasmic loss). Immunohistochemistry for p53 in conjunction with Smad4 can also provide support for a high-grade dysplasia/invasive adenocarcinoma if it demonstrates a mutant

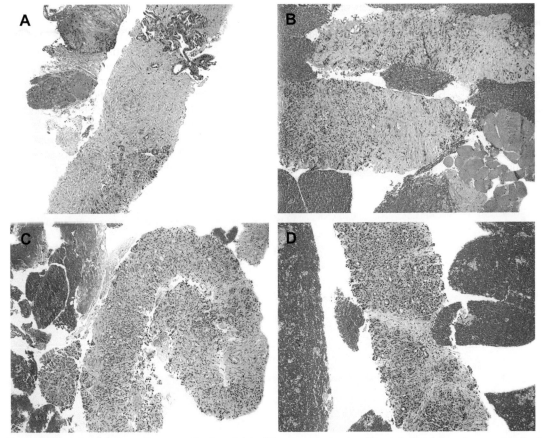

Fig. 2. (*A*) Invasive adenocarcinoma at the top right of the core contrasts with a lobule of chronic pancreatitis at the bottom right. (*B–D*) Chronic pancreatitis with maintenance of lobulated architecture.

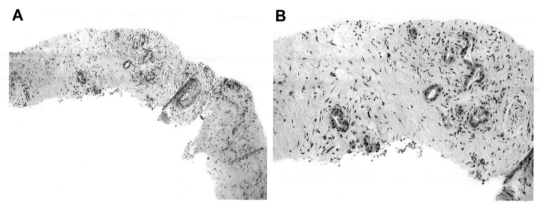

Fig. 3. Severe atrophy of pancreatic parenchyma (*A* and *B*). Note that suggestion of lobulation can still be appreciated.

phenotype (diffuse strong nuclear overexpression or complete loss of nuclear expression).

Autoimmune pancreatitis, both Type 1/IgG4-related and Type 2, can mimic adenocarcinoma, both radiographically and histologically. The classic inflammatory changes in both types, as well as elevation of IgG4+ plasma cells in Type 1, can be patchy and poorly represented on biopsy. In addition, the inflammation present may lead to significant reactive atypia in benign ducts, which can cause confusion with ductal adenocarcinoma. Although lobular architecture is retained in autoimmune pancreatitis, the inflammation and fibrosis can sometimes obscure the underlying structure (**Fig. 6**A-B). Lymphoplasmacytic inflammation, often with scattered eosinophils and the presence of fibrosis with a storiform pattern, are features seen in Type 1/IgG4-related autoimmune pancreatitis and should trigger evaluation by immunohistochemistry for IgG and IgG4. Often, a duct-centric pattern to the inflammation can be appreciated (**Fig. 6**C-D). Obliterative phlebitis is less likely to be seen on biopsy but is highly suggestive of IgG4-related disease in the presence of other specific morphologic features (**Fig. 6**E). The presence of greater than 10 IgG4+ cells per high power field on a core biopsy is supportive of but not specific for Type 1/IgG4-related autoimmune pancreatitis (**Fig. 6**F).[3] In general, an increased IgG:IgG4 ratio is often not appreciated on core biopsy and is less useful. As the elevation of IgG4+ plasma cells can be patchy, it is difficult to rule out IgG-4 related pancreatitis on a small biopsy. However, it is also uncommon to observe the constellation of characteristic findings on small biopsy, so correlation with radiographic findings (particularly the presence of systemic disease) and serum IgG4 levels is required. The presence of periductal inflammation with neutrophilic infiltration of the epithelium/neutrophilic abscesses

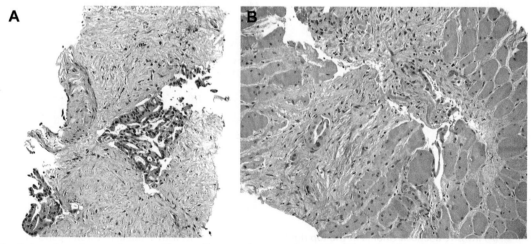

Fig. 4. Invasive adenocarcinoma with growth around a muscular artery (*A*) and within skeletal muscle (*B*).

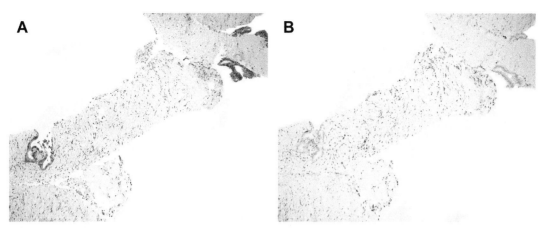

Fig. 5. (*A*) Core biopsy of a mass lesion in the pancreas showing atypical glands in a desmoplastic stroma. The architecture is suspicious for infiltration but cytologic atypia is not marked. (*B*) Immunostain for Smad4 (Dpc4) demonstrates loss of nuclear and cytoplasmic staining in the atypical glands with retained labeling in adjacent stroma, confirming an invasive adenocarcinoma.

should prompt consideration of Type 2 autoimmune pancreatitis.

Features of rare subtypes of adenocarcinoma such as adenosquamous carcinoma or undifferentiated carcinomas (including sarcomatoid carcinomas) can be difficult to appreciate on small core biopsies but their presence should be actively sought because they have the potential to change management in the neoadjuvant setting. Adenosquamous carcinomas, for example, have been shown to respond best to regimens including a platinum-based chemotherapeutic agent.[4] The presence of an aggressive morphologic component showing sarcomatoid or undifferentiated features, while not favoring a particular regimen, might influence clinical decision-making regarding neoadjuvant therapy or upfront surgery in resectable cases. Clues to squamous differentiation include distinct cell borders (which may harbor apparent cell junctions) and areas of "hard" eosinophilic cytoplasm. Immunohistochemistry for p40 can be helpful to confirm. Although a formal diagnosis of adenosquamous carcinoma requires at least 30% squamous differentiation in a broader resection sample, the presence of squamous features on a small biopsy and the possibility that they represent part of an adenosquamous carcinoma should be mentioned. If a carcinoma shows entirely squamous differentiation on a small biopsy, this still may represent sampling of an adenosquamous carcinoma, but the need to rule out the possibility of metastatic disease clinically should be communicated in the diagnosis.

When diagnosed by FNA, well-differentiated ductal adenocarcinomas should be distinguished from benign gastrointestinal contamination and

reactive atypia seen in ductal epithelium, especially in the setting of chronic pancreatitis. Knowledge of the biopsy approach and familiarity with the appearance of duodenal and gastric epithelial fragments on FNA is critical to allow one to distinguish adenocarcinoma from benign gastrointestinal contamination. Duodenal epithelium is typically encountered in the FNA of pancreatic head masses, whereas gastric epithelium is seen on FNA specimens sampling tail and body masses. Unless small, duodenal epithelial fragments contain goblet cells, which often seem as "punched out" holes at low magnification. Large fragments of gastric epithelium may preserve the three-dimensional architecture of gastric pits, although such large fragments are rarely seen. Small-to-medium-sized fragments of gastric epithelium lack goblet cells and may be seen in large numbers in procedures that fail to sample a pancreatic lesion. In these cases, an assessment for cytomorphologic features more specific to pancreatic adenocarcinoma should be performed (Box 2). If one remains uncertain whether the atypical fragments represent adenocarcinoma or gastrointestinal contamination, a definitive diagnosis of malignancy should not be made.[5]

To distinguish from reactive atypia, a diagnosis of adenocarcinoma is more readily made in a cellular specimen with a distinct population of markedly atypical cells. The presence of benign elements, such as benign acinar cells and tissue fragments, in similar or greater quantities should cause reconsideration of an adenocarcinoma diagnosis, especially if the atypia is mild. For well-differentiated adenocarcinomas, a helpful

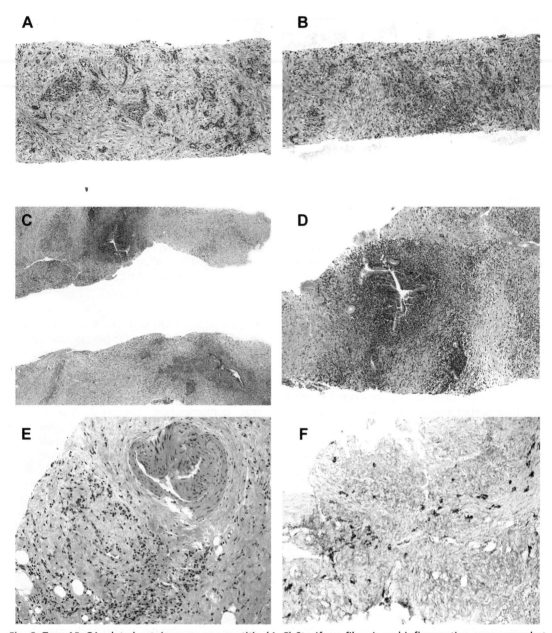

Fig. 6. Type 1/IgG4-related autoimmune pancreatitis. (*A, B*) Storiform fibrosis and inflammation may somewhat obscure the underlying lobular architecture. (*C, D*) Duct-centric lymphoplasmacytic inflammation. (*E*) Paired artery and vein with fibrosis and inflammation involving the vein wall suggestive of obliterative venulitis. (*F*) Immunostain for IgG4 showing greater than 10 cells per single HPF.

Box 2
Features supporting adenocarcinoma over chronic pancreatitis on FNA specimens

Irregularly placed nuclei within glandular fragments (drunken honeycomb)

Nuclear size variation greater than 4:1

Numerous atypical glandular/ductal fragments (vs rare numbers in pancreatitis)

Irregular nuclear contours (wrinkled nuclei and/or nuclear grooves)

Lack of granulomatous inflammation

feature is a "drunken honeycomb" architecture in which there is disorderly arrangement of nuclei within atypical tissue fragments.[6] The identification of pale nuclei with chromatin clearing and nuclear contour irregularities such as nuclear notches and/or nuclear grooves is also helpful for the diagnosis of well-differentiated adenocarcinomas. Nuclear size variation in which adjacent nuclei vary in size by 4:1 or greater is considered a specific feature but this feature may be missing in well-differentiated adenocarcinomas (**Fig. 7**). Poorly differentiated carcinomas as well as necrotic carcinomas may have numerous markedly atypical cells dispersed in the background of the specimen. Although the presence of fibroinflammatory fragments is not a specific finding, as it may represent chronic pancreatitis or areas of desmoplasia, look carefully at the edges of these fragments in an otherwise paucicellular specimen because tumor cells can sometimes cling to the edges.

Undifferentiated adenocarcinoma with osteoclast-like giant cells is typically recognized as a malignancy on FNA given the presence of overtly atypical mononuclear cells.[7] The characteristic osteoclast-like giant cells may not be as easily identified on Pap and Diff-Quik stained preparations. A potential pitfall is that the osteoclast-like cells are CD45 positive; a population of mononuclear cells may also be present and express CD45, leading to consideration of lymphoma (**Fig. 8**). The identification of the osteoclast-like giant cells may be easier on cell block preparations or core biopsies; their presence strongly suggests this diagnosis. As an aside, primary lymphoma is exceedingly rare in the pancreas.[8,9] The presence of many small lymphocytes is more likely to be sampling of a lymph node or splenule. An increased number of small lymphocytes may be seen in chronic pancreatitis; in these instances, lymphocytes will often be seen within benign acinar tissue fragments. On

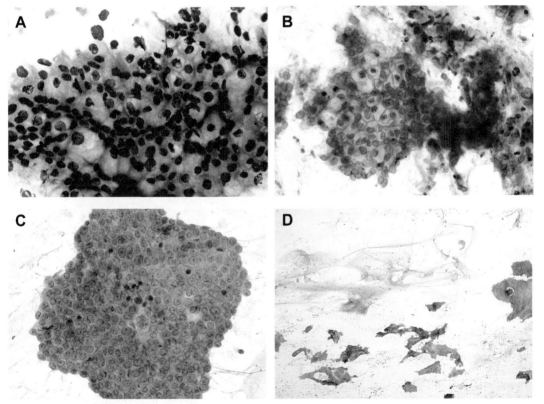

Fig. 7. Adenocarcinoma on fine needle aspiration. (*A, B*) Malignant cells contain intracytoplasmic mucin and demonstrate anisonucleosis (greater than 4:1), irregular nuclear contours, and disorganized nuclear arrangement. (*C*) A more well-differentiated fragment of adenocarcinoma from a separate patient; note the slight disorganization (drunken honeycomb) in nuclear arrangement and enlarged, pale nuclei. (*D*) Adenocarcinoma may arise within an intraductal papillary mucinous neoplasm, in which case the background may contain abundant "clean" mucin and numerous fragments with papillary architecture. Examination of cytologic features at high magnification is critical to identify features of high-grade atypia, which can represent either high-grade dysplasia or adenocarcinoma (difficult to distinguish on cytology alone).

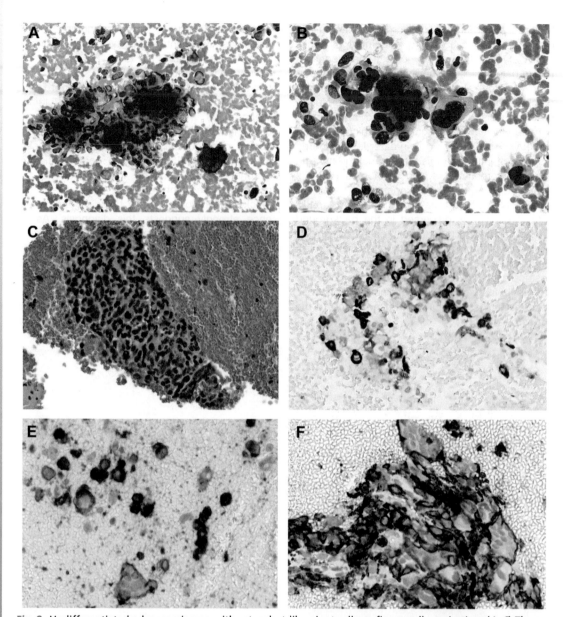

Fig. 8. Undifferentiated adenocarcinoma with osteoclast-like giant cells on fine needle aspiration. (*A–C*) The malignant cells are typically pleomorphic and may become intermixed with mononuclear cells that express CD45. One clue to the diagnosis is the presence of multinucleated osteoclast-like giant cells, which strongly suggest this entity in pancreatic lesions. (*D*) Pankeratin stains the adenocarcinoma cells but fails to stain the osteoclast-like giant cells and adjacent mononuclear cells. (*E, F*) CD45 strongly stains the osteoclast-like giant cells as well as numerous adjacent mononuclear cells; this may cause concern for lymphoma if one does not connect the presence of osteoclast-like giant cells to the possibility of an undifferentiated adenocarcinoma.

conventional smears, chromatin streaks will be seen radiating away from the fragments.

SOLID CELLULAR NEOPLASMS

PANCREATIC NEUROENDOCRINE TUMORS

Solid cellular neoplasms of the pancreas include neuroendocrine neoplasms, acinar cell carcinomas (ACCs) and solid pseudopapillary neoplasms (SPNs). Morphologic and immunophenotypic overlap between these entities can make their distinction challenging on small core biopsies. Well-differentiated pancreatic neuroendocrine tumors (PanNETs) must be distinguished from poorly differentiated neuroendocrine carcinomas (NEC) based on morphology. Grade 1 and Grade 2 PanNETs showing classic nested, trabecular, or ribbon-like growth with Ki67 proliferative indices of less than 20% are typically the most straightforward. However, the differential between Grade 3 PanNETs and NEC is a large potential pitfall on small biopsies where the recognition of classic neuroendocrine versus malignant features may be difficult, and this distinction as important clinical consequences as the treatment paradigms are quite disparate.[10] In general, Grade 3 PanNETs are more likely to have a Ki67 index of less than 50% and NECs are more likely to have Ki67 indices of greater than 50% (often in the 80%–90% range) with sheet-like, solid growth, necrosis and apoptosis. In very difficult cases, immunohistochemistry can be helpful. Frequent mutations in *DAXX* and *ATRX* genes are seen in PanNETs and loss of labeling for DAXX or ATRX proteins supports a diagnosis of PanNET.[11–13] In contrast, abnormal labeling for p53 (nuclear overexpression or complete loss), loss of Rb labeling or loss of Smad4 (Dpc4) labeling supports a diagnosis of NEC.

PanNET can also be easily confused with ACCs on small biopsy. ACCs may show a range of morphologies with areas demonstrating abundant acini formation to areas with diffuse sheet-like growth. Although granular eosinophilic cytoplasm and prominent single nucleoli are classic features of ACCs, these features can also be seen in PanNET. However, although PanNET can often be distinguished by their more amphiphilic eccentric cytoplasm and speckled "salt and pepper" chromatin, oncocytic variants of PanNET can closely mimic ACCs. In addition, acini in ACCs can mimic rosettes and pseudoglandular formations. Immunohistochemical markers of acinar differentiation are highly sensitive and specific and include BCL-10, chymotrypsin, and trypsin.[14,15] Immunolabeling for BCL-10 provides very strong, diffuse, granular cytoplasmic labeling in ACCs and is particularly useful on small biopsies. ACCs can express neuroendocrine markers and this represents a major potential pitfall on core biopsies. Synaptophysin or chromogranin labeling cannot rule out acinar differentiation, even when diffuse (Fig. 9). Although greater than 30% labeling with neuroendocrine markers meets technical criteria for a mixed acinar-neuroendocrine carcinoma, these tumors have the genomic features and clinical behavior of ACCs and are best considered subtypes of ACCs.[16] As such, the acinar differentiation should be emphasized on diagnosis.

On fine needle aspiration, PanNETs are suggested by the presence of numerous epithelioid cells widely dispersed in the background (Fig. 10). At higher magnification, the cells have eccentrically placed nuclei, which give them a plasmacytoid appearance. In the correct clinicoradiologic setting, these findings can be diagnostic of PanNET. However, confirmatory stains with neuroendocrine markers are preferred when possible. PanNETs are morphologically diverse and some may have rhabdoid morphology, which can cause diagnostic confusion.[17] PanNETs may also have "clear cell" or "lipid rich" variation in which vacuolated cytoplasm may mimic metastatic renal cell carcinoma, the most common metastasis to the pancreas.[18–20] Awareness of these various morphologies allows one to first consider a diagnosis of PanNET instead of less likely diagnoses.

Normal acinar cells are commonly misinterpreted as PanNET, as on conventional smears the cells may become singly dispersed and be seen in small fragments with acinar microarchitecture that mimics the rosette formations seen in some PanNETs (see Fig. 10). The dilemma is further complicated because the sampling of benign acinar tissue indicates the lesion of interest was not adequately sampled; thus, no other cell population may be present, leading one to believe that the cells seen are indeed lesional.[21] On conventional smears, PanNET cells tend to disperse more widely through the slide, whereas acinar tissue fragments and cells tend to align in the direction of the smear, with smaller fragments and single cells concentrated at one end of the slide. In cellular samples, acinar tissue will tend to maintain some larger fragments that have grapelike architecture; because PanNETs do not form this architecture, such a finding should cause consideration that the cells of interest may all be acinar cells and not neuroendocrine cells.

Splenules are well-circumscribed nodules and have similar imaging features as PanNETs. Thus, this history may bias one's opinion when reviewing a splenule on FNA. Such specimens contain numerous small lymphocytes, which will be individually dispersed and present in great numbers, similar to what is seen in PanNETs. However, the lymphocytes will also be present together with littoral cells in medium-to-large sized fragments. Although these fragments may be difficult to identify for inexperienced cytomorphologists, they are not seen in PanNET specimens. Lymphocyte nuclei may become crushed and streak away from these fragments in conventional smears, resembling granulomatous inflammation. Cell block preparations and core biopsies are often helpful because these H&E-stained preparations can allow for recognition of splenic tissue to those more familiar with seeing it in surgical specimens.

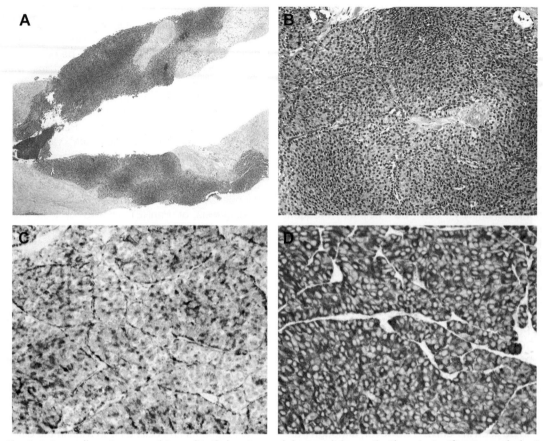

Fig. 9. Acinar cell carcinoma on biopsy (*A, B*) showing nodular to solid growth. There is significant morphologic overlap with a well-differentiated neuroendocrine tumor. Although the tumor is positive for chromogranin (*C*), it is also diffusely positive for BCL-10 (*D*), confirming an acinar phenotype.

Immunostaining with CD8 is particularly helpful because it will highlight the splenic sinusoids along with some of the mature lymphocytes (**Fig. 11**).

SOLID PSEUDOPAPILLARY NEOPLASMS

SPNs have distinctive morphologic features that can lead to fairly straightforward separation from other solid cellular neoplasms of the pancreas. These include discohesive cells with oval nuclei and delicate nuclear grooves, degenerative changes (necrosis, foamy macrophages, and cholesterol clefts) and hyaline globules. Myxoid change may be apparent around vessels with surrounding clinging epithelial cells creating the eponymous "pseudo" papillae. Diagnostic difficulty on core biopsy most often arises when sampling of an SPN shows predominantly solid areas of the tumor without degenerative changes. In these cases, morphologic overlap with PanNET can cause significant confusion as SPN can also immunolabel for synaptophysin and CD56 (**Fig. 12**). However, they typically show more

patchy cytokeratin labeling than PanNET and are characteristically negative for chromogranin.[22] The most useful immunostain on core biopsy for distinguishing SPN from PanNET is β-catenin, which will show abnormal nuclear localization in SPN (but normal membranous labeling in PanNET) due to consistent mutations in *CTNNB1*, the gene that encodes β-catenin.[23,24]

On FNA, SPN are often suggested by their distinctive clinicoradiologic features (mixed solid and cystic pancreatic mass in young women), though SPNs have been seen in unusual locations and older patients. SPN have distinctive features that, when present in the proper setting, allow for their recognition on FNA without the need for confirmatory immunostains. Prominent vessels with irregular branches should be seen; the vessels will fuse together seemingly at random, creating unusual shapes. This vascular pattern should be accompanied by monomorphic, bland neoplastic cells that line both the vessels and disperse throughout the background. Diagnostic trouble occurs when the vascular structures are

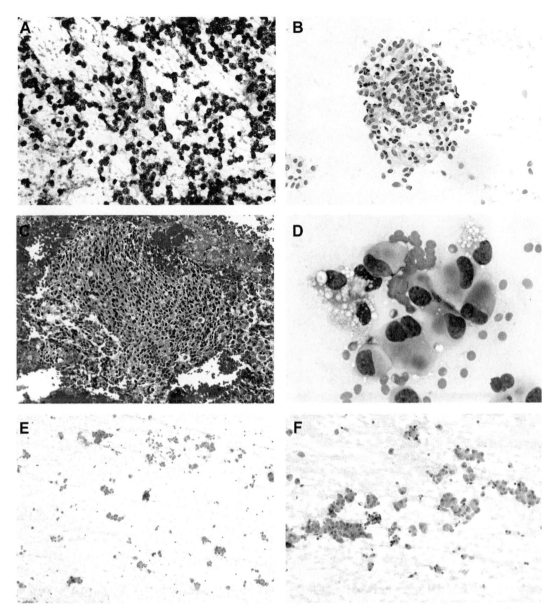

Fig. 10. PanNET on fine needle aspiration. (*A*) Neuroendocrine cells are often dispersed in conventional smears. (*B, C*) The cells typically have eccentrically placed nuclei and a "salt and pepper" chromatin pattern that is characteristic of cells with neuroendocrine differentiation. (*D*) Morphologic variations may exist that cause diagnostic dilemmas; in this case, the cells have a rhabdoid morphology. (*E, F*) The sampling of benign acinar tissue (seen here) may be confused with the sampling of a neuroendocrine tumor due to the presence of single cells, rosette structures, and a population of monotonous plasmacytoid cells. Note that in a conventional smear, benign acinar cells tend to streak in one direction, compared with the random dispersion of neuroendocrine tumor cells (seen in panel *A*).

not prominently seen, as the dispersed neoplastic cells closely resemble the neuroendocrine cells of PanNET. In such cases, immunohistochemistry can help distinguish the 2 entities. SPNs may have clear cell features, which can suggest the possibility of metastatic RCC, given that the 2 entities can also have prominent vessels (**Fig. 13**).[25]

ACINAR CELL CARCINOMA

Acinar cell carcinoma is rarely seen on FNA. More commonly, a lesion is not adequately sampled and abundant acinar tissue will be seen, causing concern for acinar cell carcinoma. Acinar cell carcinoma can look overtly malignant and mimic

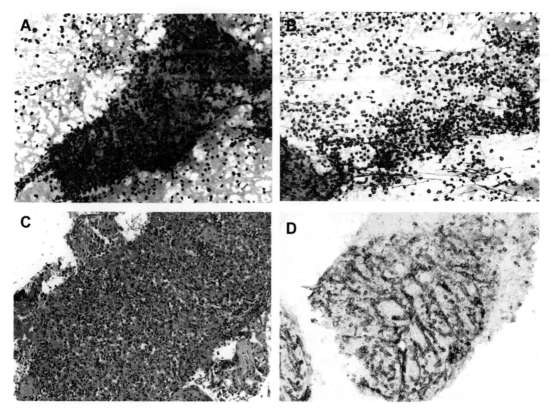

Fig. 11. Splenule on fine needle aspiration. Splenules look similar to PanNETs on imaging studies and may be an unexpected finding. (*A, B*) The sample contains numerous lymphocytes that may look like dispersed neuroendocrine cells at low magnification. Close examination will reveal these cells to be small, mature lymphocytes. (*C*) On cell block preparations, architecture resembling splenic tissue may be easier to recognize. (*D*) Staining with CD8 will highlight splenic sinusoidal cells, providing a distinctive pattern.

adenocarcinoma but ACCs cells may also seem bland and resemble benign acinar cells. In these instances, immunostaining for BCL-10 may be helpful to prove acinar differentiation. ACCs will not form the regular grapelike architecture of acinar cells; if this architecture it seen in large fragments, sampling of benign acinar tissue is much more likely than an ACCs. When considering smaller fragments, ACCs fragments will have irregular shapes and sizes compared with benign acinar tissue fragments. However, ACCs often will maintain its underlying acinar microarchitecture. In these instances, it may be very challenging to make a diagnosis of ACCs because both ACCs and benign acinar tissue will stain positively for BCL-10.[26]

As discussed above, on core biopsies, ACCs may show areas of acinar, nodular and/or solid, sheet-like growth. Prominent central nucleoli and granular eosinophilic cytoplasm are keys to the diagnosis but there is significant overlap with morphology of PanNET, particularly the oncocytic variant and a low threshold for obtaining both

neuroendocrine and acinar markers should be used.

CYSTIC LESIONS

In general, cystic lesions of the pancreas are challenging for endoscopists to target with core biopsies. Often the cores are even more fragmented and scant than is typical for solid lesions. Cyst contents only may be present (eg, macrophages, debris, and so forth), making a definitive diagnosis impossible. Contamination from the gastrointestinal tract is particularly confounding as fragments of benign gastric or duodenal mucosa can strongly mimic fragments of a neoplastic mucinous cyst such as an IPMN. Gastric contamination is the most problematic to distinguish from low-grade gastric-type IPMNs (**Fig. 14**). Intestinal-type differentiation seen in IPMNs is typically not as well developed as normal duodenal mucosa. The location of the cystic lesion can be helpful as well. Gastric contamination is most common in lesions from the body and tail,

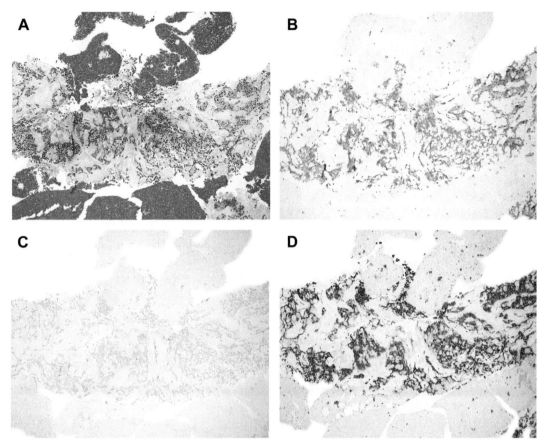

Fig. 12. (*A*) Solid-pseudopapillary neoplasm on biopsy. Note the loosely discohesive cells and myxoid and hyalinized stroma. The tumor shows immunolabeling for (*B*) synaptophysin but not chromogranin (*C*). (*D*) A β-catenin immunostain shows diffuse nuclear positivity, confirming the diagnosis of solid pseudopapillary neoplasm.

where the needle is most likely to traverse the stomach, whereas duodenal contamination is more common in lesions in the head, which are more often accessed across the duodenum.

On FNA, IPMN should be considered when either abundant extracellular thick mucin and/or atypical mucinous epithelial cells are seen in the setting of a cystic lesion (Fig. 15).[27] When a transgastric route is used to sample the lesion, contamination with foveolar epithelium may occur; it is difficult to distinguish this benign epithelium from the mucinous epithelium of IPMNs unless high-grade dysplasia is present. The presence of abundant "clean" mucin can help with the diagnosis of IPMN because "clean" mucin only contains rare macrophages, whereas the "dirty" mucin from gastrointestinal contamination will contain bacteria and granular debris. "Clean" mucin may have unusual appearances; conventional smears with abundant mucin may have a "ferning" pattern or crystalloid appearance. Ancillary tests such as cyst fluid CEA analysis as well as cyst fluid molecular analysis can

help confirm a diagnosis of IPMN, discussed in further detail elsewhere.[28,29]

The extensive presence of mucinous epithelial fragments with high-grade cytologic atypia and/or more complex papillary architecture lessens concerns over contamination but introduces additional issues in distinguishing high-grade dysplasia from detached fragments of invasive adenocarcinoma, as was mentioned earlier. Careful correlation with radiographic findings is required in this setting. If no clear solid mass is present, extensive high-grade changes can be described as representing "at least high-grade dysplasia" and if a solid component is present, a caveat that an associated invasive carcinoma cannot be excluded should be mentioned.

The morphologic features of IPMNs with high-grade dysplasia have significant overlap with invasive adenocarcinoma, and a diagnosis of "neoplastic mucinous cyst with high-grade atypia" can be rendered with a note suggesting invasive adenocarcinoma if abundant background necrosis is present.[30]

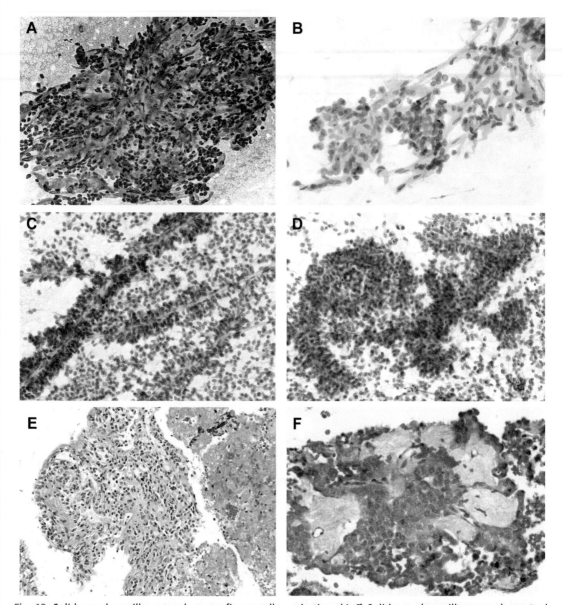

Fig. 13. Solid-pseudopapillary neoplasm on fine needle aspiration. (*A–F*) Solid-pseudopapillary neoplasms typically contain long vessels that abruptly branch and may fuse together. Monomorphic neoplastic cells are seen attached to the vessels as well as dispersed in the background. If the vascular structures are not seen, PanNET may become the main consideration in the differential diagnosis.

OTHER CYSTIC LESIONS

Additional cystic lesions commonly sampled on FNA/core biopsy include mucinous cystic neoplasms (MCNs), serous cystadenomas (SCAs), and lymphoepithelial cysts. MCNs can be separated from IPMNs based on their characteristic ovarian-type stroma, localized condensed beneath the cyst lining. However, generous biopsies demonstrating abundant ovarian stroma are not common. The stromal cells are typically positive for ER and PR. SCAs often produce particularly scant biopsy specimens but can be recognized by delicate epithelial cells with bland, round, centrally placed nuclei in a background of clear cytoplasm.[31] The glycogen-rich clear cytoplasm of SCAs can be highlighted by Periodic acid-Schiff stain and is sensitive to diastase. The combination of attenuated or squamous epithelial lining with abundant associated lymphocytes or

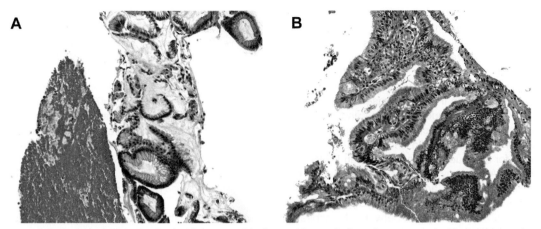

Fig. 14. (*A*) The bland, organized cuboidal-type epithelium with gastric foveolar-type mucin, likely representing gastric contamination, contrasts with the more complex papillary architecture and elongated, pencil-shaped nuclei of the likely fragment of IPMN (*B*). Focal more eosinophilic epithelial cells are suggestive of parietal cells, further supporting that the fragment represents contamination.

organized lymphoid tissue should prompt consideration of a lymphoepithelial cyst.[32,33] Of note, lymphoepithelial cysts can have elevated CEA levels and pose a pitfall in the differential with neoplastic mucinous cysts.

Pseudocysts are sometimes encountered on FNA.[34] They have no true lining and thus nonspecific cyst contents such as cystic macrophages, crystalloids, and granular debris are often aspirated. The presence of hematoidin pigment is

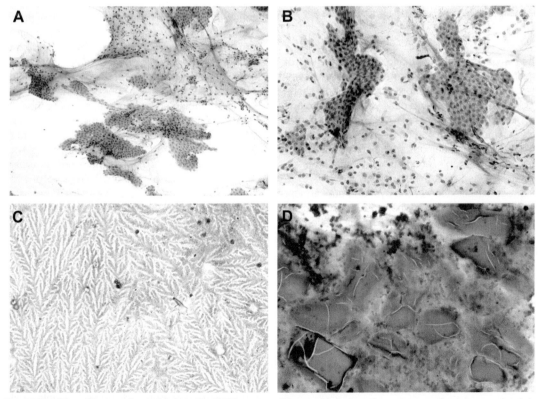

Fig. 15. IPMN on fine needle aspiration. (*A, B*) When sampling a cystic lesion, the presence of numerous glandular fragments in a background of "clean" mucin strongly suggests the sampling of a mucin-producing neoplastic cyst and is diagnostic of IPMN in the correct clinicoradiologic context. (*C, D*) Some lesions may produce acellular FNAs and contain predominantly mucin. Mucin may have various appearances and may cause a "ferning" effect when drying (*C*) or form crystals and/or crystalloids (*D*).

suggestive of a pseudocyst. A pseudocyst is often in the differential diagnosis on imaging studies. Such cases can be signed out as consistent with the clinical impression of a pseudocyst. The presence of contaminating gastric epithelium can cause diagnostic difficulty, as it may be interpreted as lining from an IPMN. Because crystalloids can also form within mucinous cysts and mucin can sometimes have a crystalloid appearance, the presence of hematoidin should cause consideration for a pseudocyst rather than an IPMN. Cyst fluid CEA and amylase levels as well as cyst fluid molecular analysis are especially helpful in these circumstances, as cytomorphology alone may not be able to distinguish between the aspiration of an IPMN versus pseudocyst in a background of gastric contamination. An additional potential pitfall is the extensive degenerative changes often seen in MCNs. Areas of MCNs can show complete denudation of the cyst lining with replacement by foamy macrophages, granulation tissue, and chronic inflammation. Sampling of such an area within an MCN may be indistinguishable from a pseudocyst. Careful examination for mucin and/ or mucinous epithelium and correlation with radiology is required.

MICROFORCEPS BIOPSIES

The evaluation of a pancreatic cyst on any type of small biopsy comes with the usual pitfalls associated with inadequate sampling of the lesional tissue (Fig. 16). For example, in a case where the cytology and fluid chemistries are not revealing as to whether a cyst is mucinous in nature, the presence of only a small strip of nonmucinous epithelium may lead to a diagnosis of a simple, nonmucinous cyst. This interpretation based on a minute biopsy would lead to incorrect classification of the cyst and subsequent patient management. Furthermore, if insufficient subepithelial stroma is obtained, the distinction between an MCN and IPMN cannot be made. Of note, the Moray microforceps biopsy was able to obtain adequate tissue to diagnose one case of MCN in a cohort of these specimens.[35] As is seen with other small biopsy specimens, benign cysts such as SCAs and pseudocyst are difficult to diagnose on microforceps biopsies because the former tends to provide scant epithelium and the latter does not have a true epithelial lining, although microforceps biopsies may allow further workup of SCA epithelium.

ANCILLARY TESTING

Ancillary molecular testing on cyst fluid can be very useful as an adjunct to FNAs and small core biopsies. Mutational analysis can help confirm cyst diagnoses and guide management in combination with histology, clinical, and radiographic features.[29,36–38] The presence of KRAS and GNAS mutations is highly sensitive for mucinous cysts (with GNAS being specific for IPMN) and the presence of alterations in TP53, p16/CDKN2A, SMAD4, PIK3CA, PTEN, and others can signal high-grade dysplasia or invasive carcinoma. VHL mutations and mutations in CTNNB1 are highly sensitive for SCAs and SPNs, respectively.[24,39]

EXTRAPANCREATIC LESIONS

When typical patterns are not recognized, it is useful to consider the possibility of unusual entities. Metastases to the pancreas are rare, and typically, the patient will have a history of malignancy. Renal cell carcinoma is the most common metastasis to the pancreas.[40] It is helpful to have a cell block preparation or small biopsy for immunohistochemical analysis in most instances. Excluding metastatic gastrointestinal adenocarcinomas and cholangiocarcinomas can be challenging due to immunoprofile overlap. Although the loss of Smad4/Dpc4 by immunohistochemistry was previously noted to be helpful for identifying ductal adenocarcinoma versus reactive ductal epithelium, caution is needed when using this finding to distinguish pancreatic ductal adenocarcinoma from other metastatic carcinomas, including ~20% of colorectal adenocarcinomas and ~15% of cholangiocarcinomas, among others.[41]

A diagnostic pitfall to keep in mind when a diagnosis of PanNET is considered is a pancreatic or peripancreatic paraganglioma.[42] The nested architecture of these neoplasms can be easily confused with the organoid architecture of PanNET. However, a clue to the diagnosis of paraganglioma is lack of cytokeratin expression in a solid cellular neoplasm showing immunolabeling for synaptophysin and chromogranin. Although PanNETs can rarely lack keratin labeling, paraganglioma should be considered in this setting. Immunolabeling with GATA3 and S-100 and/or SOX10 labeling in a sustentacular pattern provides additional support for a diagnosis of paraganglioma.[43]

Adrenal cortical tissue is sometimes sampled accidentally when an FNA procedure fails to target a pancreatic mass. The sampling of benign adrenal cortical tissue can result in a very cellular specimen with numerous dispersed single cells expressing neuroendocrine markers. This may result in the incorrect diagnosis of a PanNET. Adrenal tissue is often better recognized on H&E-stained cell block preparations and small biopsies.

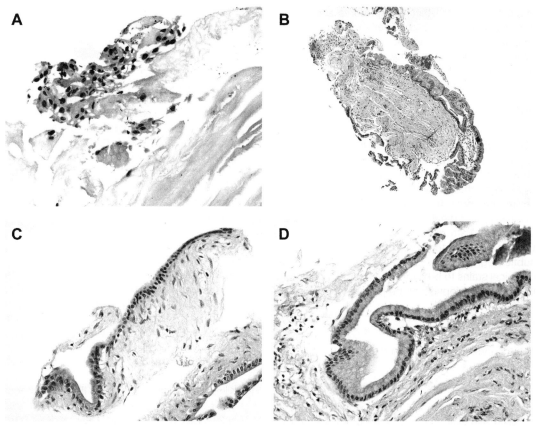

Fig. 16. Moray microforceps biopsies. (*A*) Serous cystadenoma. The epithelial cells have small, round, uniform nuclei and clear, glycogen-rich cytoplasm. (*B–D*) IPMN with low-grade dysplasia. The epithelium is mucinous with bland, basally oriented nuclei. In some biopsies of IPMNs, mucinous epithelium is only seen focally (*C*, lower left). No subepithelial ovarian-type stroma is present in any of these biopsies.

The proceduralist may report having difficulty sampling the pancreatic lesion during the procedure.

GISTs and schwannomas may form well-circumscribed masses in close relation to the pancreas and are therefore sometime sampled on FNA.[44–46] When sampled, these lesions may have a distinct population of bland spindled cells. In these instances, immunostains can be used to definitively diagnose GIST (DOG1 and c-kit positive and S-100 protein negative) or schwannoma (DOG1 and c-kit negative and S-100 protein positive). Both schwannoma and GIST may seem as a mixed population of epithelioid and spindled cells on FNA, which can cause diagnostic difficulty. Schwannomas may undergo ancient change causing markedly atypical spindle cells to be seen on FNA. Because these cases may cause a concern for sarcoma that cannot be resolved with immunohistochemical studies, it is important to list the benign diagnosis of schwannoma in the differential diagnosis. Some of these diagnostic challenges can be ameliorated on core

biopsy, where features of ancient change such as hyalinized vessels may help resolve concerns over atypical spindle cells and Antoni A and B areas and Verocay bodies may be represented.

Paragangliomas are often adjacent to the pancreas and may be mistaken for pancreatic lesions on imaging. As discussed above, these are often mistaken for well-differentiated neuroendocrine tumors on both FNA and core biopsy but a classic nested architecture and lack of cytokeratin labeling can be important diagnostic clues. A rare tumor of the periampullary region may occasionally be encountered on small biopsies labeled as "pancreas." These tumors show a triphasic growth pattern comprising epithelioid cells, spindle cells (Schwannian stroma), and ganglion cells. Most commonly these tumors are mistaken for well-differentiated neuroendocrine tumors if only the epithelioid component is sampled or the spindled stroma is not sampled because these epithelioid cells will label with cytokeratin and neuroendocrine markers. Less commonly, sampling of only the spindled stroma could lead to confusion with a schwannoma or other benign nerve sheath tumor. Thus, one should consider excluding entities such as GIST, schwannoma, paraganglioma, and gangliocytic paraganglioma when encountering unusual spindled and or/epithelioid neoplasms in the pancreas on FNA.

SUMMARY

The evaluation of small cytopathology and surgical biopsy specimens of the pancreas presents numerous diagnostic challenges. The limited nature of the samples can make identification of subtle morphologic features difficult, allowing for mimickers and pitfalls to create significant obstacles to accurate diagnoses. Here, we have provided a practical toolkit of morphologic patterns, subtle diagnostic clues and ancillary immunohistochemical stains to breakdown even the most challenging small biopsies of the pancreas.

DISCLOSURE

The authors have nothing to disclose.

REFERENCES

1. Hahn SA, Schutte M, Hoque AS, et al. DPC4, a candidate tumor suppressor gene at human chromosome 18q21. 1. Science 1996;271(5247):350–3.
2. Wilentz RE, Su GH, Le Dai J, et al. Immunohistochemical labeling for dpc4 mirrors genetic status in pancreatic adenocarcinomas: a new marker of DPC4 inactivation. Am J Pathol 2000;156(1):37–43.
3. Detlefsen S, Klöppel G. IgG4-related disease: with emphasis on the biopsy diagnosis of autoimmune pancreatitis and sclerosing cholangitis. Virchows Arch 2018;472(4):545–56.
4. Wild AT, Dholakia AS, Fan KY, et al. Efficacy of platinum chemotherapy agents in the adjuvant setting for adenosquamous carcinoma of the pancreas. J Gastrointest Oncol 2015;6(2):115.
5. Pitman MB, Layfield LJ. Guidelines for pancreaticobiliary cytology from the Papanicolaou Society of Cytopathology: a review. Cancer Cytopathol 2014; 122(6):399–411.
6. Collins JA, Ali SZ, VandenBussche CJ. Pancreatic cytopathology. Surg Pathol Clin 2016;9(4):661–76.
7. Reid MD, Muraki T, HooKim K, et al. Cytologic features and clinical implications of undifferentiated carcinoma with osteoclastic giant cells of the pancreas: an analysis of 15 cases. Cancer Cytopathol 2017;125(7):563–75.
8. Adsay NV, Andea A, Basturk O, et al. Secondary tumors of the pancreas: an analysis of a surgical and autopsy database and review of the literature. Virchows Arch 2004;444(6):527–35.
9. Salvatore JR, Cooper B, Shah I, et al. Primary pancreatic lymphoma: a case report, literature review, and proposal for nomenclature. Med Oncol 2000;17(3):237–47.
10. Tang LH, Basturk O, Sue JJ, et al. A practical approach to the classification of WHO grade 3 (G3) well differentiated neuroendocrine tumor (WD-NET) and poorly differentiated neuroendocrine carcinoma (PD-NEC) of the pancreas. Am J Surg Pathol 2016;40(9):1192.
11. Jiao Y, Shi C, Edil BH, et al. DAXX/ATRX, MEN1, and mTOR pathway genes are frequently altered in pancreatic neuroendocrine tumors. Science 2011; 331(6021):1199–203.
12. VandenBussche CJ, Allison DB, Graham MK, et al. Alternative lengthening of telomeres and ATRX/DAXX loss can be reliably detected in FNAs of pancreatic neuroendocrine tumors. Cancer Cytopathol 2017;125(7):544–51.
13. Heaphy CM, VandenBussche CJ. Prognostic biomarkers in pancreatic neuroendocrine tumors. Cancer Cytopathol 2021;129(11):841–3.
14. La Rosa S, Franzi F, Marchet S, et al. The monoclonal anti-BCL10 antibody (clone 331.1) is a sensitive and specific marker of pancreatic acinar cell carcinoma and pancreatic metaplasia. Virchows Arch 2009;454(2):133–42.
15. Klimstra DS, Heffess CS, Oertel JE, et al. Acinar cell carcinoma of the pancreas. A clinicopathologic study of 28 cases. Am J Surg Pathol 1992;16(9):815–37.
16. Nagtegaal ID, Odze RD, Klimstra D, et al. The 2019 WHO classification of tumours of the digestive system. Histopathology 2020;76(2):182.
17. Fite JJ, Ali SZ, VandenBussche CJ. Fine-needle aspiration of a pancreatic neuroendocrine tumor with prominent rhabdoid features. Diagn Cytopathol 2018;46(7):600–3.
18. Reid MD, Balci S, Saka B, et al. Neuroendocrine tumors of the pancreas: current concepts and controversies. Endocr Pathol 2014;25(1):65–79.
19. Schreiner AM, Mansoor A, Faigel DO, et al. Intrapancreatic accessory spleen: mimic of pancreatic endocrine tumor diagnosed by endoscopic ultrasound-guided fine-needle aspiration biopsy. Diagn Cytopathol 2008;36(4):262–5.
20. Conway AB, Cook SM, Samad A, et al. Large platelet aggregates in endoscopic ultrasound-guided fine-needle aspiration of the pancreas and peripancreatic region: a clue for the diagnosis of intrapancreatic or accessory spleen. Diagn Cytopathol 2013;41(8):661–72.
21. Ahmed A, VandenBussche CJ, Ali SZ, et al. The dilemma of "indeterminate" interpretations of pancreatic neuroendocrine tumors on fine needle aspiration. Diagn Cytopathol 2016;44(1):10–3.
22. Dinarvand P, Lai J. Solid pseudopapillary neoplasm of the pancreas: a rare entity with unique features. Arch Pathol Lab Med 2017;141(7):990–5.

23. Tanaka Y, Kato K, Notohara K, et al. Frequent β-catenin mutation and cytoplasmic/nuclear accumulation in pancreatic solid-pseudopapillary neoplasm. Cancer Res 2001;61(23):8401–4.

24. Abraham SC, Klimstra DS, Wilentz RE, et al. Solid-pseudopapillary tumors of the pancreas are genetically distinct from pancreatic ductal adenocarcinomas and almost always harbor β-catenin mutations. Am J Pathol 2002;160(4):1361–9.

25. Zhao P, deBrito P, Ozdemirli M, et al. Solid-pseudopapillary neoplasm of the pancreas: awareness of unusual clinical presentations and morphology of the clear cell variant can prevent diagnostic errors. Diagn Cytopathol 2013;41(10):889–95.

26. Stelow EB, Bardales RH, Shami VM, et al. Cytology of pancreatic acinar cell carcinoma. Diagn Cytopathol 2006;34(5):367–72.

27. Emerson RE, Randolph ML, Cramer HM. Endoscopic ultrasound-guided fine-needle aspiration cytology diagnosis of intraductal papillary mucinous neoplasm of the pancreas is highly predictive of pancreatic neoplasia. Diagn Cytopathol 2006;34(7):457–62.

28. Cizginer S, Turner B, Bilge AR, et al. Cyst fluid carcinoembryonic antigen is an accurate diagnostic marker of pancreatic mucinous cysts. Pancreas 2011;40(7):1024–8.

29. Springer S, Wang Y, Dal Molin M, et al. A combination of molecular markers and clinical features improve the classification of pancreatic cysts. Gastroenterology 2015;149(6):1501–10.

30. Pitman MB, Centeno BA, Daglilar ES, et al. Cytological criteria of high-grade epithelial atypia in the cyst fluid of pancreatic intraductal papillary mucinous neoplasms. Cancer Cytopathol 2014;122(1):40–7.

31. Lilo MT, VandenBussche CJ, Allison DB, et al. Serous cystadenoma of the pancreas: potentials and pitfalls of a preoperative cytopathologic diagnosis. Acta Cytol 2017;61(1):27–33.

32. Groot VP, Thakker SS, Gemenetzis G, et al. Lessons learned from 29 lymphoepithelial cysts of the pancreas: institutional experience and review of the literature. HPB 2018;20(7):612–20.

33. VandenBussche CJ, Maleki Z. Fine-needle aspiration of squamous-lined cysts of the pancreas. Diagn Cytopathol 2014;42(7):592–9.

34. Gonzalez Obeso E, Murphy E, Brugge W, et al. Pseudocyst of the pancreas: the role of cytology and special stains for mucin. Cancer Cytopathol 2009;117(2):101–7.

35. Zhang ML, Arpin RN, Brugge WR, et al. Moray micro forceps biopsy improves the diagnosis of specific pancreatic cysts. Cancer Cytopathol 2018;126(6):414–20.

36. Springer S, Masica DL, Dal Molin M, et al. A multimodality test to guide the management of patients with a pancreatic cyst. Sci Transl Med 2019;11(501):eaav4772.

37. Singhi AD, McGrath K, Brand RE, et al. Preoperative next-generation sequencing of pancreatic cyst fluid is highly accurate in cyst classification and detection of advanced neoplasia. Gut 2018;67(12):2131–41.

38. Zhang ML, Pitman MB. Practical Applications of Molecular Testing in the Cytologic Diagnosis of Pancreatic Cysts. J Mol Pathol 2021;2(1):11–22.

39. Reid MD, Choi H, Balci S, et al. Serous cystic neoplasms of the pancreas: clinicopathologic and molecular characteristics. Semin Diagn Pathol 2014;31(6):475–83.

40. Smith AL, Odronic SI, Springer BS, et al. Solid tumor metastases to the pancreas diagnosed by FNA: a single-institution experience and review of the literature. Cancer Cytopathol 2015;123(6):347–55.

41. Ritterhouse LL, Wu EY, Kim WG, et al. Loss of SMAD4 protein expression in gastrointestinal and extra-gastrointestinal carcinomas. Histopathology 2019;75(4):546–51.

42. Singhi AD, Hruban RH, Fabre M, et al. Peripancreatic paraganglioma: a potential diagnostic challenge in cytopathology and surgical pathology. Am J Surg Pathol 2011;35(10):1498–504.

43. Miettinen M, Cue PAM, Sarlomo-Rikala M, et al. GATA 3–a multispecific but potentially useful marker in surgical pathology–a systematic analysis of 2500 epithelial and non-epithelial tumors. Am J Surg Pathol 2014;38(1):13.

44. Bui TD, Nguyen T, Huerta S, et al. Pancreatic schwannoma. A case report and review of the literature. JOP 2004;5(6):520–6.

45. Yan BM, Pai RK, Dam JV. Diagnosis of pancreatic gastrointestinal stromal tumor by EUS guided FNA. JOP 2008;9(2):192–6.

46. McHugh KE, Odronic SI, Smith A, et al. Spindle cell neoplasms of the upper gastrointestinal tract, hepatobiliary tract, and pancreas by fine needle aspiration: a single institutional experience of 15 years with follow-up data. Diagn Cytopathol 2021;49(9):987–96.

Integrating Molecular Analysis into the Pathologic Evaluation of Pancreatic Cysts

Phoenix D. Bell, MD, MS*, Aatur D. Singhi, MD, PhD

KEYWORDS

• Pancreatic cystic lesion • Intraductal papillary mucinous neoplasm • Mucinous cystic neoplasm
• Serous cystadenoma

Key points

- Pancreatic cystic lesions are found in approximately 2% of the general population and are most often detected as incidental imaging findings.

- Mucinous pancreatic cysts include intraductal papillary mucinous neoplasm and mucinous cystic neoplasm. Early detection of mucinous pancreatic cysts is important as they can give rise to PDAC.

- Molecular analysis of pancreatic cyst fluid can stratify patients with pancreatic cystic lesions into those with low or high risk of progression.

Abbreviations

IPMN	intraductal papillary mucinous neoplasm
MCN	mucinous cystic neoplasm
SCA	serous cystadenoma
PDA	Cpancreatic ductal adenocarcinoma

ABSTRACT

The development of cross-sectional imaging techniques has enhanced the detection of pancreatic cystic lesions (PCLs). PCLs are found in approximately 2% of the general population, often as incidentally detected lesions on computed tomography or MRI during the evaluation of other medical conditions. Broadly, PCLs are classified as mucinous or nonmucinous. Mucinous PCLs include mucinous cystic neoplasms and intraductal papillary mucinous neoplasms. Nonmucinous PCLs include pseudocysts, serous cystadenomas, solid pseudopapillary neoplasms, and cystic pancreatic neuroendocrine tumors, as well as cystic acinar cell carcinoma, cystic degeneration of pancreatic ductal adenocarcinoma, lymphoepithelial cyst, and others.

OVERVIEW

The development of cross-sectional imaging techniques has enhanced the detection of pancreatic cystic lesions (PCLs). PCLs are found in approximately 2% of the general population,[1,2] often as incidentally detected lesions on computed tomography (CT) or magnetic resonance imaging (MRI) during the evaluation of other medical conditions. Broadly, PCLs are classified as mucinous or

---

Department of Pathology, University of Pittsburgh Medical Center, 200 Lothrop St. Pittsburgh, PA 15213, USA
* Corresponding author.
E-mail address: bellpd@upmc.edu

Surgical Pathology 15 (2022) 455–468
https://doi.org/10.1016/j.path.2022.05.009

nonmucinous. Mucinous PCLs include mucinous cystic neoplasms (MCNs) and intraductal papillary mucinous neoplasms (IPMNs). Nonmucinous PCLs include pseudocysts, serous cystadenomas (SCAs), solid pseudopapillary neoplasms (SPNs), and cystic pancreatic neuroendocrine tumors (cPanNETs), as well as cystic acinar cell carcinoma, cystic degeneration of pancreatic ductal adenocarcinoma (PDAC), lymphoepithelial cyst, and others. Frequently, PCLs are clinically indolent; however, up to 15% of mucinous cysts give rise to PDAC.[3] PDAC has a poor prognosis with a 5-year survival rate of 10%[4] and by 2030 is predicted to be the second leading cause of cancer-related death.[5] Thus, the premalignant nature of mucinous cysts emphasizes the importance of early detection and proper management of these lesions before they evolve into cancer. Current management guidelines are based on a multimodal approach that includes clinical presentation, imaging findings, cytopathologic interpretation, and serum biomarker levels. Despite the improvement of PCL management in recent years, some patients still receive under-treatment or overtreatment due to misclassification of their PCL. Recently, several studies have demonstrated the ability to detect high-grade dysplasia (HGD) and carcinoma in PCLs using molecular analysis of cyst fluid.[6] Having the ability to stratify patients with PCLs into those with low or high risk of progression has the potential to alter management and impact prognosis.

THE UTILITY OF MOLECULAR ANALYSIS IN PANCREATIC CYST MANAGEMENT

The development of molecular techniques has improved our understanding of the evolution of PDAC and its relationship to certain PCLs. PDAC arises through the progression of pancreatic intra-epithelial neoplasia (PanIN), from PanIN with low-grade dysplasia (LGD) to PanIN with HGD, and eventually to invasive carcinoma.[7] This disease progression occurs through the acquisition of genomic alterations, such as those in KRAS, CDKN2A, TP53, and SMAD4. Additional alterations such as telomere shortening and aneuploidy have also been documented.[8,9] Similar changes have been seen in mucinous cysts, including those associated with HGD and invasive carcinoma.[10] Here, the authors present the clinicopathologic findings of common PCLs including key mutations that can be detected by pancreatic cyst fluid (PCF) analysis, which may influence strategies for clinical intervention.

INTRADUCTAL PAPILLARY MUCINOUS NEOPLASM

IPMNs are the second most common pancreatic cyst, comprising up to 50% of PCLs.[1] IPMNs are grossly visible mucinous cysts that arise from the epithelial lining of the pancreatic ductal system.[11] They originate from the main pancreatic duct (main duct IPMN [MD-IPMN]), branches of the main pancreatic duct (branch duct IPMN), or both the main and branch ducts (mixed-type IPMN).[12] Their cause is unknown. IPMNs are premalignant and may show LGD or HGD.[11,13] Most IPMNs occur in adults around their seventh decade of life with a fairly equal male to female distribution.[14–16] In some cases, patients present with nonspecific abdominal pain, jaundice, nausea, or vomiting[14–17]; however, most IPMNs are incidental lesions detected on imaging.[12] The mucin produced by IPMNs accumulates and leads to main duct or branch duct dilatation, which may be seen on CT or MRI.[12] If the cyst communicates with the main pancreatic duct, this is highly predictive of an MD-IPMN.[18,19] Features that suggest HGD or carcinoma on cross-sectional imaging include cyst size greater than or equal to 30 mm, thickened cyst walls, and mural nodules.[20] On endoscopic ultrasound (EUS), the classic finding for an IPMN is mucin extravasation from the ampulla of Vater.[21] EUS-fine-needle aspiration (FNA) may be helpful when cross-sectional imaging is inconclusive. EUS-FNA findings may show mucinous epithelium present as single cells, clusters, or sheets in a background of abundant mucin. Pronounced cytologic atypia may be seen in IPMNs with HGD or associated with invasive carcinoma; however, due to variability of the ducts, sampling may miss these areas.[22,23] In addition, although these findings are consistent with a mucinous cyst, they do not distinguish between an IPMN and MCN. Cyst fluid obtained from IPMNs on EUS-FNA reflect elevated carcinoembryonic antigen (CEA) levels ($\geq$192 ng/mL) and elevated amylase.[24]

Grossly, MD-IPMNs most commonly involve the pancreatic head and show marked dilatation ($\geq$1 cm) of the main pancreatic duct, intraluminal mucin, and papillary excrescences.[25] In contrast, branch duct IPMNs do not usually show duct dilatation, and they occur as single or multiple cysts in the uncinate process and pancreatic neck.[14] Mixed-type IPMNs show features of both MD-IPMN and branch duct IPMN.[26] Microscopically, IPMNs are characterized by a neoplastic proliferation of mucinous epithelium arranged in papillae with variable degrees of cytoarchitectural atypia.[21,27] They are classified as gastric, intestinal, or pancreatobiliary type.[26,28] Most of the MD-IPMNs are intestinal type, composed of papillae with tall columnar cells with apical mucin and hyperchromatic ovoid to elongated nuclei.[26,28] Intestinal-type IPMNs are often associated with colloid carcinoma, which is characterized by mucin pools dissecting through the pancreatic parenchyma. Colloid carcinoma is less common and less aggressive than conventional/tubular PDAC.[29] Most branch duct IPMNs are gastric type, which is characterized by epithelium with tall columnar cells with abundant apical mucin, basally located small round nuclei, and occasional goblet cells. The epithelium can be flat or show fingerlike papillae.[26,28] Pancreatobiliary IPMNs are composed of cuboidal cells with amphophilic cytoplasm and enlarged round nuclei that form complex papillae. High-grade morphology is common.[26,28] IPMNs may show features of LGD indicated by hyperchromatic basally located nuclei with minimal atypia. High-grade features include nuclei with loss of polarity, nuclear stratification, increased mitoses, and prominent nucleoli, as well as architectural complexity in the form of papillae or cribriforming.[25,26]

Several management guidelines for pancreatic cysts exist that are based on various clinicopathologic factors including clinical presentation, cyst size, degree of main duct dilatation, presence or absence of an enhancing mural nodule, cytologic findings, and cancer antigen (CA) 19-9 levels.[20,30,31] In surgically fit patients, resection of an IPMN is recommended for patients with worrisome features including jaundice, new-onset diabetes, acute pancreatitis, elevated CA 19-9, an enhancing mural nodule or solid component greater than 5 mm, thickened cyst wall, main duct diameter greater than 10 mm, change in main duct caliber and atrophy, size greater than or equal to 3 to 4 cm, increase in cyst size greater than or equal to 3 to 5 mm/y, and high-grade cytology.[20,30,31] If only a few of these features are present, additional workup is generally recommended in the form of imaging or EUS-FNA to determine need for resection; however, this varies from guideline to guideline. If an IPMN with HGD is resected, the American Gastroenterological Association (AGA) guidelines recommend lifelong surveillance; however, surveillance for those with LGD is unclear.[32] If the IPMN is associated with an invasive carcinoma, the surveillance should follow the same guidelines as those used for patients with PDAC.[20,30,31] The prognosis for IPMNs depends on disease severity. Noninvasive IPMNs have an excellent prognosis with a 5-year survival rate between 90% and 100%.[33] In contrast, those associated with invasive carcinoma have reported 5-year survival rates between 31% and 60%.[15,33]

Next-generation sequencing (NGS) and whole-exome sequencing techniques have identified unique mutations in PCLs, such as IPMNs. The most well-documented mutations in IPMNs are KRAS and GNAS, which occur in 60% to 80% and 40% to 80% of cases, respectively.[34–37] Together, KRAS and/or GNAS mutations are present in 96% of IPMNs.[37] Additional studies have demonstrated IPMNs with advanced neoplasia bear CDKN2A, TP53, PTEN, PIK3CA, and SMAD4 mutations.[38–42] Other mutations with increased prevalence in IPMNs include ring finger protein (RNF43) and Kruppel-like factor 4 (KLF4). RNF43 is a transmembrane E3 ubiquitin ligase involved in the Wnt signaling pathway[9] and has been identified in up to 75% of IPMNs.[36,43] Further, inactivating mutations in RNF43 have also been documented in cases of PDAC.[9] KLF4 is a zinc finger transcription factor that, in one study, has been found in greater than 50% of IPMNs, particularly those with LGD.[44]

An example of IPMN management, including the incorporation of molecular testing, is seen in **Fig. 1**. An older male patient presented with an incidentally discovered cystic lesion in the head of the pancreas that was associated with ductal dilatation and mural nodularity (see **Fig. 1**A). Cytologic preparations obtained from EUS-FNA showed debris and small clusters of cells with enlarged hyperchromatic nuclei (see **Fig. 1**B). NGS of the PCF revealed a KRAS mutation (p.G12 V) (see **Fig. 1**C) and TP53 splice site mutation (p.A307) (see **Fig. 1**D). Together, the preoperative imaging, cytologic, and molecular findings were compatible with a mucinous cyst with HGD, thus the patient underwent a Whipple procedure. The surgical resection specimen displayed a cystic mass with large papillary excrescences in the pancreatic head (see **Fig. 1**E). Histologic sections demonstrated complex papillae lined by atypical cells with loss of polarity, nuclear enlargement, and hyperchromasia (see **Fig. 1**F), diagnostic of an IPMN with HGD.

INTRADUCTAL ONCOCYTIC PAPILLARY NEOPLASM

Intraductal oncocytic papillary neoplasm (IOPN) is an epithelial neoplasm characterized by exophytic tissue within the pancreatic ducts associated with ductal dilatation, which creates a partly cystic appearance.[45,46] IOPNs tend to be solitary neoplasms that arise in the pancreatic head. IOPNs were previously classified as an oncocytic variant of IPMN; however, recent studies demonstrating

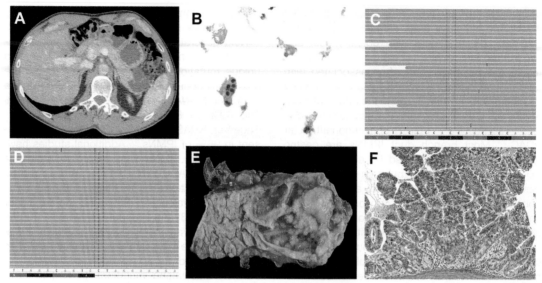

Fig. 1. IPMN with high-grade dysplasia. (*A*) Cross-sectional imaging shows a hypointense mass in the pancreatic tail. (*B*) FNA reveals rare clusters of cells with high N:C, hyperchromasia, and nuclear membrane irregularities. (*C*) NGS shows a KRAS mutation (p.G12 V) and a (*D*) TP53 splice site mutation (p.A307). (*E*) Distal pancreatectomy shows a cystic mass in the pancreatic tail with mural papillary excrescences. (*F*) Histologic examination shows complex papillae with high-grade cytologic features.

unique molecular and immunohistochemical findings have led to the reclassification of IOPNs as a distinct entity in the most recent edition of the World Health Organization Classification of Digestive System Tumors.[47] IOPNs arise in adults around the age of 60 years,[46,48,49] and there is an equal sex distribution.[46] Most IOPNs are asymptomatic, yet some patients may experience vague abdominal pain or jaundice.[48] Cross-sectional imaging studies have shown IOPNs present akin to IPMNs, as a cystic lesion associated with duct dilatation and possibly with solid/nodular areas.[50] FNA shows cells arranged in flat sheets with occasional papillae or complex branching architecture. Cells display oncocytic features with eosinophilic granular cytoplasm, round nuclei, and prominent nucleoli. Focal intracytoplasmic lumina may also be seen.[51]

Gross examination of an IOPN demonstrates a large (5–6 cm) tan-brown, friable to solid mass in the pancreatic head, associated with dilatation of the main pancreatic duct.[46,49,52] Communication with the pancreatic duct may be seen.[49] Microscopically, IOPNs have complex architecture with arborizing papillae. Delicate fibrovascular cores are covered by multiple layers of cuboidal cells with abundant eosinophilic granular cytoplasm (due to the presence of mitochondria), round nuclei, and eccentrically placed nucleoli. Intraepithelial lumina mimicking cribriform architecture may also be recognized.[46,49,53] Most IOPNs show high-grade cytologic features

including loss of polarity, hyperchromasia, increased mitoses, anisonucleosis, and prominent nucleoli.[26,52]

Despite following a more indolent course than IPMNs,[48,53] there are no published guidelines suggesting alternate management of IOPNs. Approximately 30% of IOPNs are associated with invasive carcinoma; however, the overall survival rate is better than that of conventional PDAC,[47,48] with one study demonstrating a 10-year survival rate around 94%.[48]

There are limited studies exploring the molecular alterations in IOPNs, as they were evaluated as a subtype of IPMN before reclassification. Some studies have reported the absence of KRAS, GNAS, and RNF43 mutations in IOPNs, mutations typically identified in mucinous cysts.[37,46] Mutations in ARHGAP36, ASXL1, EPHA8, and ERBB4 have also been described,[46] but these are not defining mutations. Fusions in DNAJB1-PRKACA, ATP1B1-PRKACA,[54,55] and ATP1B1-PRKACB[55] have been documented in IOPNs as well as in invasive PDAC associated with IOPNs.[55]

MUCINOUS CYSTIC NEOPLASM

MCNs comprise 10% of PCLs.[9] MCNs are mucinous cysts that arise in the pancreatic body and tail and lack communication with the pancreatic duct.[33,56,57] Most MCNs are incidental imaging findings discovered in middle-aged women during the workup for other medical concerns.[57–59] The cause is unknown, yet some have suggested that MCNs arise secondary to hormonal production from remnant ectopic ovarian tissue.[1] Similar to IPMNs, MCNs can show LGD or HGD. Up to 16% of MCNs are associated with invasive carcinoma,[56,59–61] which tend to occur in a slightly older age group.[59,60] On CT, MCNs appear as round unilocular to multilocular cysts with a thick wall and thin septations. They can range from hypo- to hyperdense depending on the presence of mucin or hemorrhage. Similarly, MRI shows heterogenous lesions with septations. In some cases, peripheral ("eggshell") calcifications may be seen, a feature highly suspicious for an associated malignancy. Other worrisome features include large size and wall thickening or mural nodules. On EUS, an MCN appears as a 1- to 2-cm fluid-filled cavity with a thin wall.[1,19] EUS-FNA specimens are frequently acellular or hypocellular. Mucinous epithelium may be present as single cells or clusters of cells in a background of abundant thick mucin. As previously mentioned, MCNs cannot be distinguished from IPMNs based on cytology alone.[22,23] Cyst fluid analysis shows elevated CEA ($\geq$192 ng/mL) and low amylase.[24]

Grossly, MCNs are solitary unilocular to multilocular cysts (average 5 cm)[60–62] that contain mucin and/or hemorrhage.[1] They have fibrous walls that may be lined by papillae or mural nodules.[21] No communication with the pancreatic duct is seen.[1,58] Macroscopic findings that suggest HGD or carcinoma include size greater than or equal to 5.0 cm, cyst wall thickening, and the presence of mural nodules/papillae.[58,59,61,62] Histologically, MCNs are typically characterized by tall columnar mucinous epithelium overlying an ovarian-type stroma.[33,63] In some cases, the epithelium is flat with cuboidal cells and scattered goblet cells. The stroma is composed of spindle cells that are positive for estrogen receptor, progesterone receptor, and inhibin,[33,56,57,64] and occasionally, luteinization is seen.[33,56] MCNs with low-grade dysplasia show minimal cytologic atypia with basally located hyperchromatic nuclei.[59] MCNs with HGD demonstrate nuclear pseudostratification, increased N:C ratios, loss of polarity, increased mitoses, and prominent nucleoli.[23,59] Complex architecture in the form of branching, budding, or cribriforming may be present.[21,25,59]

The management guidelines for MCNs depend on specific clinicopathologic features. In short, most guidelines recommend resection for MCNs greater than or equal to 30 to 40 mm that are symptomatic or that have high-risk features on imaging.[31,32] For those less than 30 to 40 mm and without a solid component or dilated PD, surveillance via MRI or EUS is suggested.[30–32] The Fukuoka guidelines recommend resection for all MCNs and limited resection for MCNs less than 4 cm and without a mural nodule.[20] Noninvasive MCN have an excellent prognosis with 5-year survival rates between 95% and 100%,[15,56,58] and complete resection is curative.[20,61,65] Thus, following resection, noninvasive MCNs do not require additional surveillance.[20,30] In contrast, the 5-year survival rate for MCNs with invasive carcinoma is around 60% to 65%,[15,58] and these patients should be followed according to the PDAC surveillance guidelines.[20,30]

Molecular analysis of MCNs shows several genetic alterations similar to IPMNs. MCNs harbor frequent KRAS mutations (35%–75%)[37,43]; however, GNAS mutations are rarely seen.[37,43,66] Similar to IPMNs with advanced neoplasia, mutations in CDKN2A and TP53 have been described in MCNs with HGD and carcinoma.[36,43,67] Further, some studies have shown that MCNs with HGD have PIK3CA mutations.[41] Lastly, RNF43 mutations have been identified in 13% to 38% of MCNs.[36,43]

SEROUS CYSTADENOMA

SCAs comprise 10% to 16% of PCLs.[68] SCAs are serous cysts that arise in the body and tail of the pancreas from centroacinar cells.[1,21] SCAs are generally solitary lesions that have no communication with the pancreatic ducts.[1] SCAs often occur in adults around their sixth decade with a female predominance.[68–70] Many patients are asymptomatic; however, some present with abdominal pain, diabetes mellitus, jaundice, nausea, and vomiting.[68,70] SCAs are associated with somatic and germline VHL (Von Hippel-Lindau) gene mutations.[71,72] When associated with VHL syndrome, diffuse involvement of the pancreas may be seen.[72,73] Rare cases of SCAs associated with invasive carcinoma have been described.[68] On CT, most SCAs appear as a well-circumscribed, multilocular lesion, with fibrous septa. The numerous cysts can impart a "honeycomb appearance," which is associated with the multicystic variant. Less often, the oligocystic variant of SCA is seen, which shows fewer larger cysts that can make it difficult to distinguish from mucinous cysts on imaging.[19,24,74] A hypodense central stellate scar is seen in up to 30% of cases.[30,73,75] On MRI, SCAs appear as hyperintense cysts with hypointense septa; a fluid signal may be seen on T2-weighted images.[75] On EUS, the multilocularity can also convey a honeycomb appearance.[70] EUS-FNA frequently results in

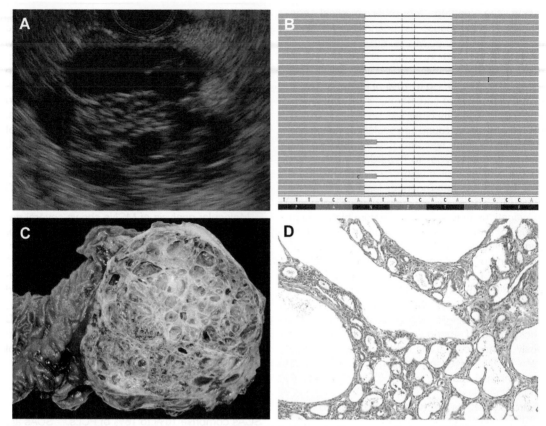

Fig. 2. Serous cystadenoma. (*A*) EUS reveals a multiloculated mass in the pancreatic head. (*B*) NGS shows a deletion in VHL (p.I151Cfs*6). (*C*) Whipple resection reveals a large lesion composed of numerous small cysts imparting a "spongelike" appearance. (*D*) Histologic sections demonstrate numerous cysts lined by small round cells with clear cytoplasm.

acellular to hypocellular specimens with hemosiderin-laden macrophages and debris. Scattered cuboidal cells in small groups or clusters may be present. The cells contain clear cytoplasm and round nuclei with smooth nuclear membranes.[23] Cyst fluid analysis reveals low CEA and amylase levels.[24]

Grossly, SCAs are solitary lesions that are classically described as having a "spongelike" or "honeycomb" appearance, secondary to the presence of multiple cysts interspersed with larger cysts. Contained within these cysts is clear, yellow serous fluid. There is no communication with the main pancreatic duct.[19] A central stellate scar may be present.[63,73,74,76] Histologically, SCAs are characterized by multiple cysts lined by a single layer of cuboidal cells with clear cytoplasm (secondary to glycogen accumulation) and round nuclei. In some cases, the epithelium may form papillae or tufts.[63,73,76]

SCAs have an excellent prognosis[68,70] and do not require surgical resection unless patients are symptomatic.[2,30] In such cases, SCAs do not require surveillance following surgery.[30]

Regarding molecular alterations, SCAs harbor unique mutations in the VHL gene on chromosome 3p25.[71,72,77] In contrast to mucinous lesions, no mutations in KRAS, GNAS, CDKN2A, or SMAD4 mutations have been described.[36,66]

An example of SCA management, including the incorporation of molecular testing, is seen in **Fig. 2**. A young woman presented with nonspecific abdominal pain, which subsequently led to imaging studies. EUS demonstrated a multiloculated lesion in the pancreatic head (see **Fig. 2**A). NGS of the PCF revealed a deletion in VHL gene (p.I151Cfs*6) (see **Fig. 2**B). Because of the symptomatic nature of this lesion, the patient underwent resection, which showed a large multiloculated mass with a "spongelike" appearance in the pancreatic head (see **Fig. 2**C). Histologic sections showed cysts lined by uniform cells with clear cytoplasm and round nuclei (see **Fig. 1**D), diagnostic of an SCA.

SOLID PSEUDOPAPILLARY NEOPLASM

SPNs make up to 3% of cystic neoplasms.[77] SPN is a malignant pancreatic tumor with indolent behavior that can present as a cystic mass secondary to degeneration.[25,78] The cause is currently enigmatic. SPNs occur throughout the pancreas, and 10% to 15% of patients develop liver or peritoneal metastasis.[79,80] Most SPNs arise in women aged between 20 and 30 years,[81,82] presenting as abdominal pain, a palpable mass with nausea/vomiting, or in some cases, they may be asymptomatic.[81,83] On cross-sectional imaging, SPNs appear as well-demarcated heterogenous masses. Similarly, EUS shows solid and cystic components.[84,85] EUS-FNA specimens are cellular and contain a monotonous population of single cells or small clusters of cells with nuclei that are round to ovoid, have fine chromatin, and have nuclear grooves. Occasionally, delicate fibrovascular stalks/papillae and myxoid material are present, which are pathognomonic for SPN.[22,23]

Grossly, SPNs are often large (4–6 cm), well-circumscribed tumors with varying degrees of solid and cystic components, hemorrhage, and necrosis.[25,56,77,79,86] Histologically, they are characterized by solid areas intermixed with cystic areas and pseudopapillary structures, composed of cells surrounding fibrovascular cores forming pseudorosettes. The cells are monomorphic and contain moderate eosinophilic cytoplasm, round to ovoid nuclei with grooves, fine chromatin, and inconspicuous nucleoli.[25,56,77,79,86] Blood, necrosis, and macrophages are often seen. Lymphovascular and perineural invasion are rare. The neoplastic cells stain positively for nuclear beta-catenin, progesterone receptor, and estrogen receptor immunostains.[25,56,77,79,86]

The primary treatment of SPNs is surgical resection.[80] Most SPNs have a good prognosis with approximately 85% to 95% of SPNs cured by surgery.[1,80,87] Following surgery, the American College of Gastroenterology guidelines recommend yearly surveillance for at least 5 years.[30] As mentioned, some patients with SPNs may have liver or peritoneal metastases, which are often amenable to surgical resection, and these patients can also have a favorable prognosis.[86,88]

In contrast to other PCLs, SPNs contain few unique mutations. Most SPNs harbor mutations in the Wnt signaling pathway, particularly point mutations in CTNNB1.[79] They also show absence of VHL mutations.[36] A subset of SPNs can also have TP53 mutations.[89] In contrast to mucinous cysts, SPNs lack mutations in KRAS, GNAS, and RNF43.[36,79]

CYSTIC PANCREATIC NEUROENDOCRINE TUMOR

PanNETs make up approximately 1% to 2% of pancreatic cancers[90] and cPanNETs make up 5% to 19% of PanNETs.[24,91–94] The cystic nature of these lesions is not well understood. It is unclear whether they arise secondary to necrosis of solid pNEN (ie, via cystic degeneration) or are a unique subtype of NETs, as they show different behavior than their solid counterparts.[21,95] cPanNETs can occur sporadically or arise in patients with multiple endocrine neoplasm (MEN) syndrome.[92,95] cPanNETs most commonly arise in the body or tail of the pancreas and are usually nonfunctioning.[95–97] They occur in individuals in their fifth decade with an equal sex distribution.[96,97] Presenting symptoms include nonspecific abdominal pain, weight loss, pancreatitis, or a palpable mass.[92] Radiologically, cPanNETs may appear solid, cystic, or have mixed solid and cystic areas. In some cases, CT highlights septations[98] or peripheral enhancement.[94] Similarly, on EUS, cPanNETs have a heterogenous appearance,[99,100] thus FNA is key in the diagnosis.[30] FNA demonstrates nonmucinous fluid with scattered single cells and loose clusters of cells with round to oval nuclei, eccentrically placed, and coarse "salt and pepper" chromatin.[23,94] Cyst fluid analysis shows low amylase levels.[24]

Grossly, cPanNETs typically range from 1 to 5 cm[92,94,101]; however, cPanNETs up to 17 cm have been documented.[97] In contrast to solid PanNETs, cPanNETs are often larger.[93,97] cPanNETs are unilocular and contain clear, straw-colored, or serosanguinous fluid.[21,94,101] No communication with the pancreatic duct is seen. Histologically, cPanNETs are characterized by a cystic space lined by fibrosis and surrounded by neuroendocrine cells.[97] The neuroendocrine cells are monotonous with round to oval nuclei with moderate cytoplasm and coarse stippled ("salt and pepper") chromatin.[21,94] The neoplastic cells stain positively for synaptophysin and chromogranin immunostains.[92,94,97]

cPanNETs are more indolent than solid PanNETs[95,102] with overall survival rates between 87% and 100%.[96] According to the European guidelines for PCL management, surgical resection is recommended for cPanNETs greater than or equal to 20 mm, whereas surveillance is suggested for those less than 20 mm, that are asymptomatic, and that have no worrisome features.[31,95] In 2021, Maggino and colleagues examined 263 cPanNETs and found that lymph node involvement on imaging, age greater than 65 years, preoperative size greater than 2 cm, and pancreatic duct dilation were independently associated with aggressive behavior,[101] thus their findings also support the surveillance recommendations proposed by the European guidelines.

Solid PanNETs have several well-known genetic mutations. PanNETs harbor germline MEN1 mutations found in patients with MEN1 syndrome, but somatic MEN1 mutations have also been described.[103] Mutations in 2 tumor suppressor genes (TSGs) involved in chromatin remodeling have been documented and include DAXX (death domain-associated protein) and ATRX (alpha thalassemia/mental retardation X-linked).[104] Mutations in these genes lead to loss of protein expression and alternative lengthening of telomeres.[90,103,104] De Wilde and colleagues[104] evaluated ATRX and DAXX expression in PanNETs from patients with MEN1 and showed that, when compared with the intact ATRX and DAXX expression found in microadenomas, the PanNETs that demonstrated loss of ATRX and/or DAXX were larger (≥3 cm); thus they concluded that these

mutations occur late in disease progression. In 2018, Chou and colleagues[90] evaluated ATRX and DAXX loss by immunohistochemistry on tissue microarrays from PNENs and found that ATRX loss was associated with poor overall survival, suggesting the incorporation of ATRX into routine practice. Lastly, alterations in genes involved in the mTOR pathway have also been detailed.[103] Despite the mutations identified in solid PanNETs, there are no studies specifically documenting similar mutations in cPanNETs.

An example of cPanNET management, including the incorporation of molecular testing, is seen in Fig. 3. A middle-aged female presented with nonspecific abdominal pain. EUS revealed a solid mass in the pancreatic tail with a central cystic component (see Fig. 3A). NGS demonstrated a deletion in MEN1 (pG.483Afs*81), compatible with a cPanNET (see Fig. 3B). The patient underwent surgical resection, which showed a large mass in the pancreatic head with solid and cystic components and a central area of hemorrhage (see Fig. 1C). Histologic sections revealed

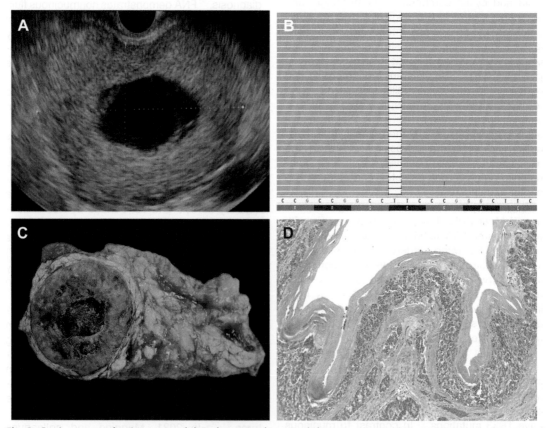

Fig. 3. Cystic neuroendocrine tumor. (*A*) Endoscopic ultrasound shows a mass in the pancreatic tail with central cyst formation. (*B*) NGS shows an MEN1 mutation (p.G483Afs*81). (*C*) Whipple resection reveals a large tan-brown mass with solid central cystic area with hemorrhage. (*D*) Histologic examination shows the cyst is lined by fibrosis and surrounded by a monotonous population of cells forming pseudorosettes.

a cystic area lined by fibrosis and surrounded by a monotonous population of small round cells forming pseudorosettes (see **Fig.** 3D), diagnostic of a cPanNET.

PSEUDOCYST

Pseudocysts make up approximately 80% of PCLs.[1] Pseudocysts most commonly arise as a complication of acute pancreatitis, chronic pancreatitis, or trauma.[105,106] In adult men, pseudocysts are most commonly caused by alcohol use, whereas in younger men/women they are more commonly secondary to biliary disease (obstruction secondary to stenosis or stones) or trauma.[25,106] Patients often present with abdominal pain, but they may be asymptomatic. Pancreatitis is caused by pancreatic enzymes that are released from a compromised pancreatic duct, which leads to fat necrosis and inflammation within the pancreatic parenchyma. When the areas of fat necrosis are resorbed, pseudocysts develop. The cysts appear as localized/walled-off areas of pancreatic tissue without epithelium and that contain pancreatic enzymes, such as amylase, and necrotic debris.[105] Regarding imaging, the diagnosis of a pseudocyst can be quite challenging, as it can mimic both premalignant cysts and malignant lesions. On CT, pseudocysts appear as a round unilocular fluid-filled cyst that can range in thickness. Some cases may show changes of adjacent pancreatitis, and when correlated with clinical history of pancreatitis, these findings strongly support a pseudocyst.[24,107] On MRI, pseudocysts demonstrate a fluid-filled cyst that may appear bright on T2-weighted images.[107] EUS shows a unilocular cyst, whereas EUS-FNA reveals scattered inflammatory cells, necrosis, blood, and lacks epithelial cells.[22,23] Cyst fluid expresses elevated amylase and low CEA.[24]

Grossly, pseudocysts are unilocular with a thick cyst wall that may contain debris or blood. A connection to the pancreatic duct is seen. Histologically, pseudocysts have a fibrous pseudocapsule, lack an epithelial lining, and are often associated with fat necrosis, inflammation, and granulation tissue. In some cases, the adjacent stroma may show increased cellularity.[25,106,108]

Most pseudocysts resolve spontaneously; however, some patients may require supportive treatment such as intravenous fluids, analgesics, or antiemetics. If a pseudocyst is symptomatic, infected, bleeding, or causing obstruction, then it should be drained, either via endoscopic transmural drainage, percutaneous catheter drainage, or open surgery.[107] As pseudocysts carry no risk of malignancy, follow-up is not needed after resection.[30]

In contrast to the previously discussed PCLs, pseudocysts do not demonstrate any unique molecular alterations, thus the management is based on clinical history, imaging, and FNA findings.

THE IMPACT OF MOLECULAR ANALYSIS ON PANCREATIC CYST LESION MANAGEMENT

Several groups have evaluated the impact of NGS of cyst fluid on the clinical management of PCLs. In 2016 Singhi and colleagues[109] conducted a study to assess the accuracy of the AGA guidelines in detecting advanced neoplasia. They studied 225 patients with pancreatic cysts who underwent EUS-FNAs from January 2014 to May 2015, assessing clinical findings, EUS features, cytopathology results, CEA analysis, and molecular alterations (KRAS, GNAS, VHL, TP53, PIK3CA, and PTEN). They found that the guidelines outlined by the AGA identified advanced neoplasia with 62% sensitivity, 79% specificity, 57% positive predictive value (PPV), and 82% negative predictive value (NPV). In comparison, the new management approach proposed by this group, which incorporated molecular testing, detected advanced neoplasia with 100% sensitivity, 90% specificity, 79% PPV, and 100% NPV. Later, in 2018, Singhi and colleagues[6] prospectively analyzed DNA alterations in 626 PCF specimens from 595 patients and correlated these findings with clinical history, imaging findings, and follow-up data. *KRAS/GNAS* mutations were identified in 56 of IPMNs and 3 of MCNs, which resulted in a sensitivity and specificity of 89% and 100% for mucinous PCLs. When *KRAS* and *GNAS* mutations were combined with mutations in *TP53*, *PIK3CA*, and *PTEN*, the calculated sensitivity and specificity was 89% and 100% for cysts with HGD or invasive carcinoma. These sensitivities and specifies were higher compared with those seen with imaging findings suspicious for advanced neoplasia, including the presence of a mural nodule (42% sensitivity, 74% specificity) and duct dilatation (32% sensitivity, 94% specificity). They were also higher than those seen with malignant cytopathology findings (32% sensitivity, 98% specificity). In 2019, Springer and colleagues developed CompCyst, a supervised machine learning technique that used clinical history, imaging findings, cyst fluid molecular alterations, and biochemical markers to guide management of PCLs. Regarding molecular alterations, this group evaluated mutations, loss of heterozygosity of chromosome regions containing TSGs known to be involved in specific cyst types, aneuploidy, and two protein markers (CEA and VEGF). The Comp-Cyst approach was compared to conventional PCL management. Their results showed that KRAS and GNAS were the most frequent mutations in IPMNs and MCNS (*KRAS*: 76% IPMNs, 35% MCNs and *GNAS*: 56% IPMNs, 2% MCNs). Further, *RNF43* mutations were identified in 39% of IPMNs and 13% of MCNs. When integrating these findings with the aforementioned CompCyst factors, they found that more than 50% of the patients underwent unnecessary surgery if conventional management was followed versus the CompCyst approach. Each of these studies demonstrates the utility of incorporating molecular techniques into PCL management to improve patient management, including decreasing morbidity and potentially improving survival.

CLINICS CARE POINTS

- IPMNs have mutations in KRAS and GNAS, which occur in 60-80% and 40-80% of cases, respectively.

- MCNs harbor frequent KRAS mutations (35-75%);however, GNAS mutations are rarely seen.

- Alterations in TP53, SMAD4 and the mTOR genes are associated with high grade dysplasia and early invasive adenocarcinoma from a mucinous cyst.

- Several studies have demonstrated that the incorporation of molecular analysis into pancreatic cyst management, increases the sensitivity and specificity for detecting advanced neoplasia, when compared to conventional cyst management.

SUMMARY

PCLs harbor unique mutations that can help guide patient management. In terms of high-risk lesions, mucinous cysts (MCNs and IPMNs) have the highest risk of malignant potential. Although mutations in KRAS and GNAS are found in these lesions, it is more difficult to identify mutations associated with areas of HGD or invasive carcinoma (TP53, CDKN2A, and SMAD4), as these mucinous cysts are quite heterogeneous. In concert with the challenge of identifying cysts at risk of progression is determining which patients should undergo molecular testing of their PCF and how these techniques can best be incorporated into management guidelines. Further, additional DNA studies, as well as RNA expression and proteomic studies, are needed to better understand the molecular profiles of PCLs.

REFERENCES

1. Brugge WR. Diagnosis and management of cystic lesions of the pancreas. J Gastrointest Oncol 2015;6(4):375–88.
2. Singhi AD, Nikiforova MN, McGrath K. DNA testing of pancreatic cyst fluid: is it ready for prime time? Lancet Gastroenterol Hepatol 2017;2(1):63–72.
3. Singhi AD, Koay EJ, Chari ST, et al. Early Detection of Pancreatic Cancer: Opportunities and Challenges. Gastroenterology 2019;156(7):2024–40.
4. Siegel RL, Miller KD, Jemal A. Cancer statistics. CA Cancer J Clin 2020;70(1):7–30.
5. Rahib L, Wehner MR, Matrisian LM, et al. Estimated Projection of US Cancer Incidence and Death to 2040. JAMA Netw Open 2021;4(4):e214708.
6. Singhi AD, McGrath K, Brand RE, et al. Preoperative next-generation sequencing of pancreatic cyst fluid is highly accurate in cyst classification and detection of advanced neoplasia. Gut 2018; 67(12):2131–41.
7. Amato E, Molin MD, Mafficini A, et al. Targeted next-generation sequencing of cancer genes dissects the molecular profiles of intraductal papillary neoplasms of the pancreas. J Pathol 2014;233(3): 217–27.
8. Macgregor-Das AM, Iacobuzio-Donahue CA. Molecular pathways in pancreatic carcinogenesis. J Surg Oncol 2013;107(1):8–14.
9. Fischer CG, Wood LD. From somatic mutation to early detection: insights from molecular characterization of pancreatic cancer precursor lesions. J Pathol 2018;246(4):395–404.
10. Goggins M, Overbeek KA, Brand R, et al. Management of patients with increased risk for familial pancreatic cancer: updated recommendations from the International Cancer of the Pancreas Screening (CAPS) Consortium. Gut 2020;69(1): 7–17.
11. Basturk O, Hong SM, Wood LD, et al. A Revised Classification System and Recommendations From the Baltimore Consensus Meeting for Neoplastic Precursor Lesions in the Pancreas. Am J Surg Pathol 2015; 39(12):1730–41.
12. Yoon JG, Smith D, Ojili V, et al. Pancreatic cystic neoplasms: a review of current recommendations for surveillance and management. Abdom Radiol (NY) 2021;46(8):3946–62.
13. Tanaka M. Intraductal Papillary Mucinous Neoplasm of the Pancreas as the Main Focus for Early Detection of Pancreatic Adenocarcinoma. Pancreas 2018;47(5):544–50.

14. Sohn TA, Yeo CJ, Cameron JL, et al. Intraductal papillary mucinous neoplasms of the pancreas: an updated experience. Ann Surg 2004;239(6): 788–97, [discussion: 797-9].

15. Crippa S, Castillo CF, Salvia R, et al. Mucin-producing neoplasms of the pancreas: an analysis of distinguishing clinical and epidemiologic characteristics. Clin Gastroenterol Hepatol 2010; 8(2):213–9.

16. Schnelldorfer T, Sarr MG, Nagorney DM, et al. Experience with 208 resections for intraductal papillary mucinous neoplasm of the pancreas. Arch Surg 2008;143(7):639–46 ; discussion 646.

17. Suzuki Y, Atomi Y, Sugiyama M, et al. Cystic neoplasm of the pancreas: a Japanese multiinstitutional study of intraductal papillary mucinous tumor and mucinous cystic tumor. Pancreas 2004;28(3): 241–6.

18. Jacobson BC, Baron TH, Adler DG, et al. ASGE guideline: The role of endoscopy in the diagnosis and the management of cystic lesions and inflammatory fluid collections of the pancreas. Gastrointest Endosc 2005;61(3):363–70.

19. Sarno A, Tedesco G, De Robertis R, et al. Pancreatic cystic neoplasm diagnosis: Role of imaging. Endosc Ultrasound 2018;7(5):297–300.

20. Tanaka M, Castillo CF, Adsay V, et al. International consensus guidelines 2012 for the management of IPMN and MCN of the pancreas. Pancreatology 2012;12(3):183–97.

21. Adsay NV. Cystic lesions of the pancreas. Mod Pathol 2007;20:S71–93.

22. Bellizzi AM, Stelow EB. Pancreatic cytopathology: a practical approach and review. Arch Pathol Lab Med 2009;133(3):388–404.

23. Pitman MB, Deshpande V. Endoscopic ultrasound-guided fine needle aspiration cytology of the pancreas: a morphological and multimodal approach to the diagnosis of solid and cystic mass lesions. Cytopathology 2007;18(6):331–17.

24. Brugge WR, Lewandrowski K, Lee-Lewandrowski E, et al. Diagnosis of pancreatic cystic neoplasms: a report of the cooperative pancreatic cyst study. Gastroenterology 2004; 126(5):1330–6.

25. Basturk O, Coban I, Adsay NV. Pancreatic cysts: pathologic classification, differential diagnosis, and clinical implications. Arch Pathol Lab Med 2009;133(3):423–38.

26. Kloppel G, Basturk O, Schlitter AM, et al. Intraductal neoplasms of the pancreas. Semin Diagn Pathol 2014;31(6):452–66.

27. Hruban RH, Goggins M, Parsons J, et al. Progression model for pancreatic cancer. Clin Cancer Res 2000;6(8):2969–72.

28. Furukawa T, Kloppel G, Adsay NV, et al. Classification of types of intraductal papillary-mucinous neoplasm of the pancreas: a consensus study. Virchows Arch 2005;447(5):794–9.

29. Adsay NV, Pierson C, Sarkar F, et al. Colloid (mucinous noncystic) carcinoma of the pancreas. Am J Surg Pathol 2001;25(1):26–42.

30. Elta GH, Enestvedt BK, Sauer BG, et al. ACG Clinical Guideline: Diagnosis and Management of Pancreatic Cysts. Am J Gastroenterol 2018; 113(4):464–79.

31. European Study Group on Cystic Tumours of the, P., European evidence-based guidelines on pancreatic cystic neoplasms. Gut 2018;67(5):789–804.

32. Vege SS, Ziring B, Jain R, et al. American gastroenterological association institute guideline on the diagnosis and management of asymptomatic neoplastic pancreatic cysts. Gastroenterology 2015;148(4):819–22, [quiz: 12-3].

33. Zamboni G, Hirabayashi K, Castelli P, et al. Precancerous lesions of the pancreas. Best Pract Res Clin Gastroenterol 2013;27(2):299–322.

34. Nikiforova MN, Khalid A, Fasanella KE, et al. Integration of KRAS testing in the diagnosis of pancreatic cystic lesions: a clinical experience of 618 pancreatic cysts. Mod Pathol 2013;26(11): 1478–87.

35. Singhi AD, Wood LD. Early detection of pancreatic cancer using DNA-based molecular approaches. Nat Rev Gastroenterol Hepatol 2021;18(7):457–68.

36. Wu J, Jiao Y, Molin MD, et al. Whole-exome sequencing of neoplastic cysts of the pancreas reveals recurrent mutations in components of ubiquitin-dependent pathways. Proc Natl Acad Sci U S A 2011;108(52):21188–93.

37. Wu J, Matthaei H, Maitra A, et al. Recurrent GNAS mutations define an unexpected pathway for pancreatic cyst development. Sci Transl Med 2011;3(92):92ra66.

38. Pea A, Yu J, Rezaee N, et al. Targeted DNA Sequencing Reveals Patterns of Local Progression in the Pancreatic Remnant Following Resection of Intraductal Papillary Mucinous Neoplasm (IPMN) of the Pancreas. Ann Surg 2017;266(1):133–41.

39. Kanda M, Sadakari Y, Borges M, et al. Mutant TP53 in duodenal samples of pancreatic juice from patients with pancreatic cancer or high-grade dysplasia. Clin Gastroenterol Hepatol 2013;11(6): 719–30.e5.

40. Schonleben F, Qiu W, Ciau NT, et al. PIK3CA mutations in intraductal papillary mucinous neoplasm/ carcinoma of the pancreas. Clin Cancer Res 2006;12(12):3851–5.

41. Garcia-Carracedo D, Chen ZM, Qiu W, et al. PIK3CA mutations in mucinous cystic neoplasms of the pancreas. Pancreas 2014;43(2):245–9.

42. Rosenbaum MW, Jones M, Dudley JC, et al. Next-generation sequencing adds value to the

preoperative diagnosis of pancreatic cysts. Cancer Cytopathol 2017;125(1):41–7.

43. Springer S, Masica DL, Molin MD, et al. A multimodality test to guide the management of patients with a pancreatic cyst. Sci Transl Med 2019;11(501).

44. Fujikura K, Hosoda W, Felsenstein M, et al. Multiregion whole-exome sequencing of intraductal papillary mucinous neoplasms reveals frequent somatic KLF4 mutations predominantly in low-grade regions. Gut 2021;70(5):928–39.

45. Jyotheeswaran S, Zotalis G, Penmetsa P, et al. A newly recognized entity: intraductal "oncocytic" papillary neoplasm of the pancreas. Am J Gastroenterol 1998;93(12):2539–43.

46. Basturk O, Tan M, Bhanot U, et al. The oncocytic subtype is genetically distinct from other pancreatic intraductal papillary mucinous neoplasm subtypes. Mod Pathol 2016;29(9):1058–69.

47. Basturk O, et al. Pancreatic intraductal oncocytic papillary neoplasm. In: Arends MJ, et al, editors. WHO classification of tumours: digestive system tumours. Lyon (France): International Agency for Research on Cancer; 2019. p. 315–6.

48. Wang T, Askan G, Adsay V, et al. Intraductal oncocytic papillary neoplasms: clinical-pathologic characterization of 24 cases, with an emphasis on associated invasive carcinomas. Am J Surg Pathol 2019;43(5):656–61.

49. Adsay NV, Adair CF, Heffess CS, et al. Intraductal oncocytic papillary neoplasms of the pancreas. Am J Surg Pathol 1996;20(8):980–94.

50. D'Onofrio M, De Robertis R, Martini PT, et al. Oncocytic Intraductal Papillary Mucinous Neoplasms of the Pancreas: Imaging and Histopathological Findings. Pancreas 2016;45(9):1233–42.

51. Reid MD, Stallworth CR, Lewis MM, et al. Cytopathologic diagnosis of oncocytic type intraductal papillary mucinous neoplasm: Criteria and clinical implications of accurate diagnosis. Cancer Cytopathol 2016;124(2):122–34.

52. Liszka L, Pajak J, Zielinska-Pajak E, et al. Intraductal oncocytic papillary neoplasms of the pancreas and bile ducts: a description of five new cases and review based on a systematic survey of the literature. J Hepatobiliary Pancreat Sci 2010; 17(3):246–61.

53. Basturk O, Chung SM, Hruban RH, et al. Distinct pathways of pathogenesis of intraductal oncocytic papillary neoplasms and intraductal papillary mucinous neoplasms of the pancreas. Virchows Arch 2016;469(5):523–32.

54. Vyas M, Hechtman JF, Zhang Y, et al. DNAJB1-PRKACA fusions occur in oncocytic pancreatic and biliary neoplasms and are not specific for fibrolamellar hepatocellular carcinoma. Mod Pathol 2020;33(4):648–56.

55. Singhi AD, Wood LD, Parks E, et al. Recurrent Rearrangements in PRKACA and PRKACB in Intraductal Oncocytic Papillary Neoplasms of the Pancreas and Bile Duct. Gastroenterology 2020; 158(3):573–82.e2.

56. Reddy RP, Smyrk TC, Zapiach M, et al. Pancreatic mucinous cystic neoplasm defined by ovarian stroma: demographics, clinical features, and prevalence of cancer. Clin Gastroenterol Hepatol 2004; 2(11):1026–31.

57. Thompson LD, Becker RC, Przygodski RM, et al. Mucinous cystic neoplasm (mucinous cystadenocarcinoma of low-grade malignant potential) of the pancreas: a clinicopathologic study of 130 cases. Am J Surg Pathol 1999;23(1):1–16.

58. Yamao K, Yanagisawa A, Takahashi K, et al. Clinicopathological features and prognosis of mucinous cystic neoplasm with ovarian-type stroma: a multiinstitutional study of the Japan pancreas society. Pancreas 2011;40(1):67–71.

59. Crippa S, Salvia R, Warshaw AL, et al. Mucinous cystic neoplasm of the pancreas is not an aggressive entity: lessons from 163 resected patients. Ann Surg 2008;247(4):571–9.

60. Keane MG, Shamali A, Nilsson LN, et al. Risk of malignancy in resected pancreatic mucinous cystic neoplasms. Br J Surg 2018;105(4):439–46.

61. Gil E, Choi SH, Choi DW, et al. Mucinous cystic neoplasms of the pancreas with ovarian stroma. ANZ J Surg 2013;83(12):985–90.

62. Jang KT, Park SM, Basturk O, et al. Clinicopathologic characteristics of 29 invasive carcinomas arising in 178 pancreatic mucinous cystic neoplasms with ovarian-type stroma: implications for management and prognosis. Am J Surg Pathol 2015;39(2):179–87.

63. Compagno J, Oertel JE. Microcystic adenomas of the pancreas (glycogen-rich cystadenomas): a clinicopathologic study of 34 cases. Am J Clin Pathol 1978;69(3):289–98.

64. Ridder GJ, Maschek H, Flemming P, et al. Ovarianlike stroma in an invasive mucinous cystadenocarcinoma of the pancreas positive for inhibin. A hint concerning its possible histogenesis. Virchows Arch 1998;432(5):451–4.

65. Sarr MG, Carpenter HA, Prabhakar LP, et al. Clinical and pathologic correlation of 84 mucinous cystic neoplasms of the pancreas: can one reliably differentiate benign from malignant (or premalignant) neoplasms? Ann Surg 2000;231(2):205–12.

66. Springer S, Wang Y, Molin MD, et al. A combination of molecular markers and clinical features improve the classification of pancreatic cysts. Gastroenterology 2015;149(6):1501–10.

67. Conner JR, Marino-Enriquez A, Mino-Kenudson M, et al. Genomic Characterization of Low- and High-Grade Pancreatic Mucinous

Cystic Neoplasms Reveals Recurrent KRAS Alterations in "High-Risk" Lesions. Pancreas 2017; 46(5):665–71.

68. Jais B, Rebours V, Malleo G, et al. Serous cystic neoplasm of the pancreas: a multinational study of 2622 patients under the auspices of the International Association of Pancreatology and European Pancreatic Club (European Study Group on Cystic Tumors of the Pancreas). Gut 2016;65(2):305–12.

69. Khashab MA, Shin EJ, Amateau S, et al. Tumor size and location correlate with behavior of pancreatic serous cystic neoplasms. Am J Gastroenterol 2011;106(8):1521–6.

70. Kimura W, Moriya T, Hirai I, et al. Multicenter study of serous cystic neoplasm of the Japan pancreas society. Pancreas 2012;41(3):380–7.

71. Vortmeyer AO, Lubensky IA, Fogt F, et al. Allelic deletion and mutation of the von Hippel-Lindau (VHL) tumor suppressor gene in pancreatic microcystic adenomas. Am J Pathol 1997;151(4):951–6.

72. Mohr VH, Vortmeyer AO, Zhuang Z, et al. Histopathology and molecular genetics of multiple cysts and microcystic (serous) adenomas of the pancreas in von Hippel-Lindau patients. Am J Pathol 2000;157(5):1615–21.

73. Reid MD, Choi H, Balci S, et al. Serous cystic neoplasms of the pancreas: clinicopathologic and molecular characteristics. Semin Diagn Pathol 2014; 31(6):475–83.

74. Warshaw AL, Compton CC, Lewandrowski K, et al. Cystic tumors of the pancreas. New clinical, radiologic, and pathologic observations in 67 patients. Ann Surg 1990;212(4):432–43 ; discussion 444-5.

75. Choi JY, Kim MJ, Lee JY, et al. Typical and atypical manifestations of serous cystadenoma of the pancreas: imaging findings with pathologic correlation. AJR Am J Roentgenol 2009;193(1):136–42.

76. Shorten SD, Hart WR, Petras RE. Microcystic adenomas (serous cystadenomas) of pancreas. A clinicopathologic investigation of eight cases with immunohistochemical and ultrastructural studies. Am J Surg Pathol 1986;10(6):365–72.

77. Kosmahl M, Pauser U, Peters K, et al. Cystic neoplasms of the pancreas and tumor-like lesions with cystic features: a review of 418 cases and a classification proposal. Virchows Arch 2004; 445(2):168–78.

78. Klimstra DS, Wenig BM, Heffess CS. Solid-pseudopapillary tumor of the pancreas: a typically cystic carcinoma of low malignant potential. Semin Diagn Pathol 2000;17(1):66–80.

79. Abraham SC, Klimstra DS, Wilentz RE, et al. Solid-pseudopapillary tumors of the pancreas are genetically distinct from pancreatic ductal adenocarcinomas and almost always harbor beta-catenin mutations. Am J Pathol 2002;160(4):1361–9.

80. Salvia R, et al. Clinical and biological behavior of pancreatic solid pseudopapillary tumors: report on 31 consecutive patients. J Surg Oncol 2007; 95(4):304–10.

81. Papavramidis T, Papavramidis S. Solid pseudopapillary tumors of the pancreas: review of 718 patients reported in English literature. J Am Coll Surg 2005;200(6):965–72.

82. Tjaden C, Hassenpflug M, Hinz U, et al. Outcome and prognosis after pancreatectomy in patients with solid pseudopapillary neoplasms. Pancreatology 2019;19(5):699–709.

83. Matsunou H, Konishi F. Papillary-cystic neoplasm of the pancreas. A clinicopathologic study concerning the tumor aging and malignancy of nine cases. Cancer 1990;65(2):283–91.

84. De Robertis R, Marchegiani G, Catania M, et al. Solid Pseudopapillary Neoplasms of the Pancreas: Clinicopathologic and Radiologic Features According to Size. AJR Am J Roentgenol 2019;213(5): 1073–80.

85. Cantisani V, Mortele KJ, Levy A, et al. MR imaging features of solid pseudopapillary tumor of the pancreas in adult and pediatric patients. AJR Am J Roentgenol 2003;181(2):395–401.

86. Cai Y, Ran X, Xie S, et al. Surgical management and long-term follow-up of solid pseudopapillary tumor of pancreas: a large series from a single institution. J Gastrointest Surg 2014;18(5):935–40.

87. Estrella JS, Li L, Rashid A, et al. Solid pseudopapillary neoplasm of the pancreas: clinicopathologic and survival analyses of 64 cases from a single institution. Am J Surg Pathol 2014;38(2):147–57.

88. Hao EIU, Hwang HK, Yoon DS, et al. Aggressiveness of solid pseudopapillary neoplasm of the pancreas: A literature review and meta-analysis. Medicine (Baltimore) 2018;97(49):e13147.

89. Kim SA, Kim MS, Kim MS, et al. Pleomorphic solid pseudopapillary neoplasm of the pancreas: degenerative change rather than high-grade malignant potential. Hum Pathol 2014;45(1):166–74.

90. Chou A, Itchins M, de Reuver PR, et al. ATRX loss is an independent predictor of poor survival in pancreatic neuroendocrine tumors. Hum Pathol 2018;82:249–57.

91. Ahrendt SA, Komorowski RA, Demeure MJ, et al. Cystic pancreatic neuroendocrine tumors: is preoperative diagnosis possible? J Gastrointest Surg 2002;6(1):66–74.

92. Bordeianou L, Vagefi PA, Sahani D, et al. Cystic pancreatic endocrine neoplasms: a distinct tumor type? J Am Coll Surg 2008;206(6):1154–8.

93. Nakashima Y, Ohtsuka T, Nakamura S, et al. Clinicopathological characteristics of non-functioning cystic pancreatic neuroendocrine tumors. Pancreatology 2019;19(1):50–6.

94. Singhi AD, Chu LC, Tatsas AD, et al. Cystic pancreatic neuroendocrine tumors: a clinicopathologic study. Am J Surg Pathol 2012;36(11):1666–73.

95. Zhu JK, Wu D, Xu JW, et al. Cystic pancreatic neuroendocrine tumors: A distinctive subgroup with indolent biological behavior? A systematic review and meta-analysis. Pancreatology 2019; 19(5):738–50.

96. Koh YX, Chok AY, Zheng HL, et al. A systematic review and meta-analysis of the clinicopathologic characteristics of cystic versus solid pancreatic neuroendocrine neoplasms. Surgery 2014;156(1): 83–96.e2.

97. Goh BKP, L.L.P.J.O., Tan YM, et al. Clinico-pathological features of cystic pancreatic endocrine neoplasms and a comparison with their solid counterparts. EJSO 2006;32:3.

98. Kawamoto S, Johnson PT, Shi C, et al. Pancreatic neuroendocrine tumor with cystlike changes: evaluation with MDCT. AJR Am J Roentgenol 2013; 200(3):W283–90.

99. Lee DW, Kim MK, Kim HG. Diagnosis of pancreatic neuroendocrine tumors. Clin Endosc 2017;50(6): 537–45.

100. Ishii T, Katanuma A, Toyonaga H, et al. Role of Endoscopic Ultrasound in the Diagnosis of Pancreatic Neuroendocrine Neoplasms. Diagnostics (Basel) 2021;11(2).

101. Maggino L, Schmidt A, Kading A, et al. Reappraisal of a 2-Cm cut-off size for the management of cystic pancreatic neuroendocrine neoplasms: a multicenter international study. Ann Surg 2021;273(5):973–81.

102. Partelli S, Cirocchi R, Crippa S, et al. Systematic review of active surveillance versus surgical management of asymptomatic small non-functioning pancreatic neuroendocrine neoplasms. Br J Surg 2017;104(1):34–41.

103. Jiao Y, Shi C, Edil BH, et al. DAXX/ATRX, MEN1, and mTOR pathway genes are frequently altered in pancreatic neuroendocrine tumors. Science 2011;331(6021):1199–203.

104. de Wilde RF, Heaphy CM, Maitra A, et al. Loss of ATRX or DAXX expression and concomitant acquisition of the alternative lengthening of telomeres phenotype are late events in a small subset of MEN-1 syndrome pancreatic neuroendocrine tumors. Mod Pathol 2012;25(7):1033–9.

105. Kim YH, Saini S, Sahani D, et al. Imaging diagnosis of cystic pancreatic lesions: pseudocyst versus nonpseudocyst. Radiographics 2005;25(3): 671–85.

106. Kloppel G. Chronic pancreatitis of alcoholic and nonalcoholic origin. Semin Diagn Pathol 2004; 21(4):227–36.

107. Habashi S, Draganov PV. Pancreatic pseudocyst. World J Gastroenterol 2009;15(1):38–47.

108. Kloppel G. Acute pancreatitis. Semin Diagn Pathol 2004;21(4):221–6.

109. Singhi AD, Zeh HJ, Brand RE, et al. American Gastroenterological Association guidelines are inaccurate in detecting pancreatic cysts with advanced neoplasia: a clinicopathologic study of 225 patients with supporting molecular data. Gastrointest Endosc 2016;83(6):1107–17.e2.

The Cytomorphologic and Molecular Assessment of Bile Duct Brushing Specimens

Caroline F. Hilburn, MD[a,b], Martha B. Pitman, MD[a,b],*

KEYWORDS

- Cytology • Bile duct brushing • Stricture • Molecular analysis • FISH • NGS

Key points

- Biliary duct brushing cytology is the standard of care for the assessment of bile duct strictures but suffers from low sensitivity for the detection of a high-risk stricture.
- Pathologic diagnosis of strictures is optimized by integration of cytomorphology and molecular analysis with fluorescence in situ hybridization or next-generation sequencing.
- Bile duct cancers are genetically heterogeneous, requiring analysis of multiple gene panels to increase sensitivity.
- Actionable mutations with targeted therapies are currently in clinical trials for the treatment of patients with bile duct cancer.

ABSTRACT

Biliary duct brushing cytology is the standard of care for the assessment of bile duct strictures but suffers from low sensitivity for the detection of a high-risk stricture. Pathologic diagnosis of strictures is optimized by integration of cytomorphology and molecular analysis with fluorescence in situ hybridization or next-generation sequencing. Bile duct cancers are genetically heterogeneous, requiring analysis of multiple gene panels to increase sensitivity. Using molecular analysis as an ancillary test for bile duct brushing samples aids in the identification of mutations that support the diagnosis of a high-risk stricture as well as the identification of actionable mutations for targeted therapies currently in clinical trials for the treatment of patients with bile duct cancer.

OVERVIEW

Bile duct strictures are a common diagnostic challenge. Potential etiologies range from benign to malignant, with most of the malignant biliary strictures resulting from pancreaticobiliary or ampullary carcinomas.[1] Patients with primary sclerosing cholangitis (PSC) are at high risk for developing cholangiocarcinoma (CCA), and early detection of high-grade dysplasia is the goal of surveillance. Despite the high morbidity (40%–50%) and mortality (3%–6%) rates, surgical resection, sometimes with neoadjuvant chemotherapy, is the treatment of choice: liver transplant for CCA and pancreaticoduodenectomy for distal bile duct adenocarcinoma.[2,3] For patients with PSC, liver transplant has shown favorable outcomes for certain forms of CCA.[3] Despite these interventions, the 5-year survival rate for all-stage extrahepatic CCA is approximately 10%.[4] Given the adverse prognosis of pancreaticobiliary carcinomas, early and definitive surgical intervention is the goal of evaluating and surveilling bile duct strictures, but the substantial morbidity and mortality of surgery mean that specificity takes priority over sensitivity in the diagnosis of malignancy. Current diagnostic strategies are multidisciplinary and involve the integration of demographic and clinical data, laboratory data, radiology, endoscopic imaging, and histologic and cytopathologic specimens.

a Department of Pathology, Massachusetts General Hospital, 55 Fruit Street, Boston, MA 02114, USA;
b Harvard Medical School, Boston, USA
* Corresponding author.
E-mail address: mpitman@partners.org

Surgical Pathology 15 (2022) 469–478
https://doi.org/10.1016/j.path.2022.05.002
1875-9181/22/© 2022 Elsevier Inc. All rights reserved.

Benign strictures compose approximately 30% of bile duct strictures that come to clinical attention and are most frequently caused by post-surgical changes, PSC, stones, pancreatitis, and IgG4-related sclerosing cholangitis.[5,6] Patients present with incidental findings such as elevated bilirubin, alkaline phosphatase, or gamma-glutamyltransferase on routine laboratories or with jaundice. The management is then centered around the restoration of bile flow, frequently relying on endoscopic stent placement and surveillance. In PSC patients, the elevated risk of malignancy requires a careful investigation of any stricture for evolving or established malignancy, especially if a mass is present.

The cytologic analysis is the current foundation of the diagnostic algorithm, but with the historically low sensitivity of cytology for the detection of malignancy,[7,8] ancillary testing with fluorescence in situ hybridization (FISH) and, more recently, molecular analysis with next-generation sequencing (NGS), has become increasingly valuable adjuncts to the evaluation process.[9–12] The molecular analysis builds on the diagnostic value of cytomorphology to reduce the number of indeterminate results and provide prognostic and therapeutically relevant results.

SAMPLING TECHNIQUES OF BILE DUCT STRICTURES

The most common sampling method of a strictured bile duct is brushing the strictured duct during endoscopic retrograde cholangio pancreatography (ERCP). The bile duct is cannulated, and a brush is passed back and forth across the stricture through the endoscope under fluoroscopy.[13] Brushing a strictured pancreatic duct is performed in a similar manner.[14,15] Multiple techniques for increasing the diagnostic yield of ERCP brushings have been investigated, including the use of repeat brushing and larger, more angled brushes, with mixed results.[16] Small tissue biopsies can be acquired using a forceps biopsy or a 19G or 22G needle.[17–20] ERCP forceps biopsy and brush cytology show comparable diagnostic performance.[19] Although ERCP provides therapeutic value by re-establishing bile drainage and diagnostic value by providing specimens of biliary epithelium for analysis, it is not an entirely benign procedure and has a high-complication rate, including the risk of cholangitis, pancreatitis, and bleeding.[21] In this setting, it is crucial to maximizing the diagnostic value of material obtained via ERCP.

TISSUE TRIAGE OF BILE DUCT BRUSHING SPECIMENS AND SMALL TISSUE BIOPSIES

Bile duct brushings (BDBs) can be smeared directly onto glass slides, but rinsing the brush in preservative solutions for liquid-based processing optimizes cellular preservation with less mechanical artifact of the cells, which already have an instrumentation effect from the procedure alone. Tissue in a liquid medium provides cells for cell-block preparation or ancillary studies, such as FISH and NGS. Molecular analysis of the cells from BDBs is an important factor in improving the sensitivity of the test.[9–11,22] Rapid on-site evaluation adds no value as the interpretation does not affect the procedure, and preservation of material for ancillary testing is preferred. Small tissue biopsies should be placed directly into formalin for routine histologic processing and can provide additional material for molecular analysis.

CYTOMORPHOLOGY OF BILE DUCT BRUSHINGS

Normal ductal cells present as flat, cohesive sheets with even nuclear spacing and cells displaying round to oval nuclei, inconspicuous nucleoli, fine chromatin, and non-mucinous cytoplasm (**Fig. 1**). Overtly malignant ductal cells show features of malignancy typical of what is seen on fine needle aspiration biopsy, including

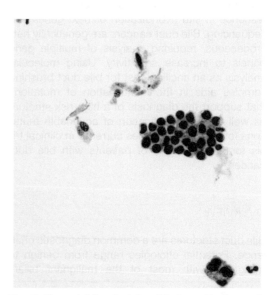

Fig. 1. Normal bile ductal epithelium. Benign cells present as flat, cohesive sheets with even nuclear spacing and display round to oval nuclei, inconspicuous nucleoli, fine chromatin, and non-mucinous cytoplasm.

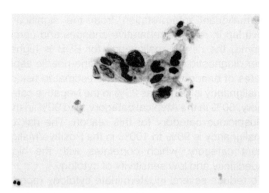

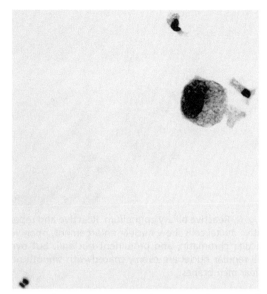

Fig. 2. Adenocarcinoma. Sheets of cells with a loss of the benign "honeycomb" pattern ("drunken honeycomb"), enlarged nuclei with anisonucleosis of 3 to 4:1, increased nuclear/cytoplasmic ratio, coarse chromatin with clumping, loss of polarity, and mucinous cytoplasm are features of overt malignancy.

sheets of cells with a loss of the benign "honeycomb" pattern ("drunken honeycomb"), enlarged nuclei with anisonucleosis of 3 to 4:1, increased nuclear/cytoplasmic ratio, intact single atypical cells, coarse chromatin with clumping, flattened nuclei, cell-in-cell arrangement, nuclear molding, and mucinous cytoplasm (Fig. 2).[23–29] These criteria for malignancy become relatively easy to identify when compared with benign ductal cells (Fig. 3) and when accompanied by single malignant cells in the background (Fig. 4),[30] but the real-life application of the criteria is extremely difficult to implement because of the overlapping features of malignancy and atypical repair, frequently resulting in atypical and suspicious interpretations rather than a definitive diagnosis of malignancy (Fig. 5).[23,25,31] A review of NGS-positive BDBs showed that more than 50% of cancers were undetected on cytology.[29] A high threshold for malignancy comes from the significant reactive atypia known to occur from

Fig. 4. Adenocarcinoma. Single intact malignant cells support the diagnosis. Note the difference between the large malignant cell with mucinous cytoplasm next to the small benign columnar ductal cell to the right.

underlying inflammatory conditions, stones, and indwelling stents. Reactive and reparative ductal cells can show nuclear enlargement, nucleoli, irregular nuclei, increased nuclear to cytoplasmic ratio, and even coarse chromatin (Fig. 6). Even with small tissue biopsies, the diagnosis of malignancy is a challenge (Fig. 7).[32,33] In particular, patients with PSC have increased rates of false-negative and false-positive results based on

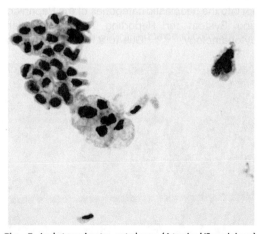

Fig. 5. Indeterminate cytology (Atypical/Suspicious). When scant in nature, the deceptively low nuclear to cytoplasmic ratio of malignant cells (bottom, right cluster of five cells), coupled with subtle nuclear atypia, makes a definitive diagnosis challenging.

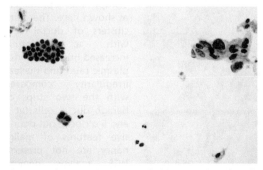

Fig. 3. Adenocarcinoma and benign ductal cells. When seen together, the distinction between benign and malignant cells is more obvious.

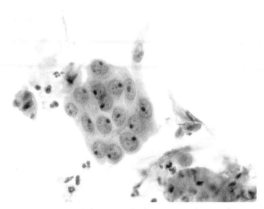

Fig. 6. Reactive biliary epithelium. Reactive and reparative ductal cells show nuclear enlargement, open vesicular chromatin, and prominent nucleoli, but overall regular nuclei are evenly spaced with smooth nuclear membranes.

cytology alone, underscoring the need for ancillary testing.[34]

REPORTING BILE DUCT BRUSHING CYTOLOGY AND RISK OF MALIGNANCY

A definitive diagnosis of dysplasia and even malignancy in BDB specimens is extremely difficult due to overlapping features with marked reactive "atypia" from inflammatory conditions, such as PSC, stones and indwelling stents,[29] and little data are available for accurate cytologic classification of intraductal bile duct neoplasms. As such, most cytologic interpretations fall in the Benign/Negative, Positive/Malignant, or conventional indeterminate categories of Atypical and Suspicious and not into the neoplastic categories of the Papanicolaou System for Reporting Pancreaticobiliary Cytopathology.[18,35,36] Due to a high threshold for

a malignant interpretation from the significant overlap in reactive/reparative changes and carcinoma, the risk of malignancy for BDB is higher per diagnostic category than for fine-needle aspirates of pancreatic masses. The estimated risk of malignancy is as high as 25% in the Negative category, 50% in the Atypical category, and 90% in the Suspicious category for this reason. The risk of malignancy is 96% to 100% in the Positive/Malignant category, which correlates with the high specificity and low sensitivity of cytology.[10,34,37,38] To reduce several indeterminate cytology reports and to improve diagnostic yield, genetic analysis of the cells in BDB samples has gained significant traction in recent years.

FLUORESCENCE IN-SITU HYBRIDIZATION

FISH is performed using a commercial kit (UroVysion probe set, Abbott Molecular Incorporated, Des Plaines, IL) that uses DNA probes to label the pericentromeric regions of chromosomes 3, 7, and 17, and the chromosomal band 9p21p.[39] A normal FISH result has two colors for each probe resulting in a benign interpretation. Trisomy 7 is frequently observed in inflammatory strictures, which is supported by the absence of elevated serum cancer antigen 19-9 (CA 19-9) values as well as the absence of a mass lesion.[40] Four signals for each probe (tetrasomy) generally reflect high cell turnover, more likely from repair and regeneration and are seldom associated with cancer.[41] Polysomy reflects gains of two or more of the four probes in at least five cells and signifies chromosomal instability (**Fig. 8**), which, in the setting of a new stricture, is considered a positive test result with a 95% specificity for malignancy.[42,43] Given that only approximately 80% of all pancreaticobiliary malignancies demonstrate

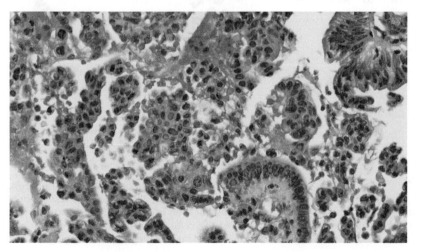

Fig. 7. Bile duct biopsy. Forceps biopsies can disrupt the epithelium, as shown here. There are clusters of ductal cells with a uniformly increased nuclear to cytoplasmic ratio and nuclear irregularity compared with the two strips of benign ductal cells (at 1 and 5 o'clock), but definitive features of malignancy are not present. NGS analysis demonstrated *KRAS* and *ARID1A* mutations supporting neoplasia.

Fig. 8. Fluorescent in situ hybridization of benign and malignant bile duct cells. Using pericentromeric regions of chromosomes 3, 7, and 17 and the chromosomal band 9p21p, the normal FISH result has two colors for each probe resulting in a benign interpretation. Polysomy reflects gains of two or more of the four probes in at least five cells and signifies chromosomal instability supporting malignancy. (Reproduced *with permission from* Gores, G.J. (2014), Addressing unmet clinical needs: FISHing for bile duct cancer. Cancer Cytopathology, 122: 789-790.)

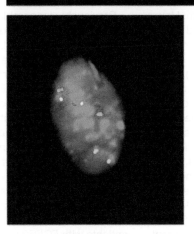
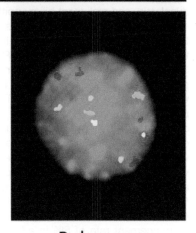

CEP 3 CEP 7 CEP 17 LSI 9p21

Disomy
2 copies of each probe

Polysomy
Gain of 2 or more probes

chromosomal instability resulting in aneuploidy, FISH analysis has inherently limited sensitivity.[44] A FISH test depends the cells analyzed that requires highly skilled technicians with excellent morphologic skills. For patients with PSC, whereby cytomorphology can be challenging, serial polysomy on FISH analysis has been associated with a high risk of malignancy.[41] The more subjective nature of DNA analysis coupled with the detailed mutational analysis offered by NGS has led to an interest in this technique as an ancillary test for BDB over FISH.

MUTATIONAL ANALYSIS AND NEXT-GENERATION SEQUENCING

Many testing modalities have been used to collect molecular data from bile duct specimens, including immunohistochemistry, single-gene PCR assays, microarray, and NGS. This accumulation of data has improved our understanding of biliary tract malignancies and the diagnostic yield of cytology specimens and provided promising prognostic information and therapeutic targets. Given that many biliary cytology specimens are characterized by low total cellularity and heterogeneous cell populations, NGS provides an ideal method of running multiple gene panels on limited specimens while maintaining analytical sensitivity.[11] In addition, NGS can be performed on multiple specimen types, including brush biopsies, fine-needle aspirates, and biopsy specimens,

allowing streamlined integration into pre-existing specimen workflows.

Biliary malignancies have a diverse set of associated genetic alterations and frequently show multiple genetic alterations within one specimen, with the most common being *TP53* (16%-40%), *KRAS* (5%–42%), *SMAD4* (3%–21%), *HER2* (11%–17%), *NF1* (6%), *ARID1A* (2%–12%), *ERBB3* (5%), *CDKN2A* (2%), and *PIK3CA* (4%–5%).[4,11,45] Among these, *TP53*, *SMAD4*, and *CDKN2A* are considered late mutations and are highly specific for malignancy.[29]

The most commonly reported mutated gene in biliary tumors is *TP53*, reported in 26% of cases and is strongly correlated with malignant, invasive disease.[10,45] Immunohistochemical staining of biliary brush cytology specimens and biopsies for p53, the protein product of *TP53*, shows over expression of the p53 protein in many cases, with increased expression in poorly differentiated cases.[16,38]

Within the cell-proliferation associated pathways, the RAS/RAF cell proliferation axis and the PI3K/AKT/mTOR cell survival signaling axis are frequently altered in CCA.[46] *KRAS* is an oncogene that is commonly mutated in biliary neoplasia and has been identified in premalignant, as well as in invasive processes, requiring caution when present as the only detected mutation, as it may indicate the presence of an incidental precursor lesion.[10]

Tumor suppressor genes are also involved. *PTEN* is a negative regulator of the PI3K/AKT signaling axis, acting as a tumor suppressor gene. In one microarray study of 221 patients, PTEN expression was no different between normal, dysplastic, and malignant biliary epithelium. However, low PTEN expression was associated with a lower overall survival time, especially in combination with activation of AKT or mTOR.[47]

Fibroblast growth factor receptor (FGFR) family proteins participate in malignant transformation via activation of the RAS, JAK/STAT, and PI3K pathways. The FGFR alterations are the most common in intrahepatic CCAs but occasionally occur in extrahepatic biliary malignancies as well.[48] Specifically, FGFR2 alterations, with various translocation partners, are promising therapeutic candidates. One study that identified FGFR2 rearrangements with FISH break-apart probes and RNA sequencing found an FGFR2 rearrangement rate of 5% in advanced/recurrent biliary tract cancers. These patients showed a distinct clinical phenotype, with overall younger age and hepatitis virus positivity.[49]

A recent study by Dudley and colleagues showed that NGS was as good as, if not better than, FISH for the detection of a high-risk stricture harboring at least high-grade dysplasia.[10] Singhi and colleagues have shown how the integration of a cancer-specific NGS panel (BiliSeq) with cytology into the routine evaluation of bile duct strictures increases the detection of malignant strictures, particularly in patients with PSC. Within the cohort of 220 patients, the BiliSeq panel had a sensitivity and specificity of 73% and 100%, respectively, with the combination of cytomorphologic evaluation and BiliSeq testing leading to a sensitivity of 95% and a specificity of 68%.[11] These results strongly support the integration of NGS testing into the routine diagnostic process for new biliary strictures.

Coupled with an understanding of the molecular drivers of carcinogenesis, molecular data show promise as a source of prognostic information. In one study, genetic alterations, including mutations in ARID1A and KRAS and under-expression of MUC17, were associated with decreases in overall survival and disease-free survival.[45] In another study of 221 patients with extrahepatic CCA, PTEN expression was associated with poor patient outcomes. TP53 mutations have likewise been associated with poor survival in biliary tract tumors.[48] The improved overall survival is seen in patients with biliary tract cancer harboring FGFR alterations. Within the FGFR family, FGFR2 mutations are the most common in biliary tract malignancies.[50] These patients are commonly younger, more likely to be female, present with earlier stage disease, and have better overall

survival than those without FGFR alterations, even accounting for the benefits of targeted therapy.[48]

Previously, inoperable biliary carcinoma was treated with stenting and chemotherapy, including gemcitabine and cisplatin. Biliary tract malignancies are a genetically heterogeneous group with a tendency for the rapid development of therapeutic resistance, which creates a challenging environment for targeted therapy. However, there are many trials currently underway working to identify actionable mutational targets for directed therapy.[46] Among biliary malignancies, approximately 13% to 68% harbor at least one potentially targetable alteration, with the most common arising in the RAS signaling pathway.[4,11,51] Now, multiple phase-3 trials targeting biliary tract malignancies are underway, including pemigatinib for patients with FGFR2 rearranged CCA and ivosidenib for patients with IDH1 mutated CCA.[10,52] Trials targeting EGFR and VEGF mutations have shown modest, partial responses.[4] In addition, patients with CCA have been included in trials of targeted therapies for the following molecular targets: PD-1, HER2/neu, PD-L1, CTLA4, and MEK1/2.[51]

Biliary cytology specimens that are negative for malignancy may provide valuable genetic information that can shed light on a patient's ongoing risk of CCA. Specifically, polymorphisms in genes involved in DNA repair, cellular protection, and immunologic surveillance, including MTHFR, TYMS, GSTO1, XRCC1, ABCC2, CYP1A2, NAT2, KLRK1, MICA, and PTGS2, are known to influence the risk of CCA.[46] Overall, germline mutations in genes known to confer increased cancer risk, including DNA mismatch repair genes and BRCA, have been described in 11% of biliary tract carcinomas.[45]

The diagnostic process surrounding biliary strictures likely remain highly multidisciplinary, with molecular data supporting cytomorphologic and laboratory findings, such as carcinoembryonic antigen (CEA) and CA-19.9. Correlations between genetic alterations detected via NGS and cytomorphologic findings have been reported, supporting the strong connection between molecular data and morphologic findings in biliary cytology. In one study, increased single cells and architectural disarray were noted in NGS-positive specimens. Nuclear changes, including increased nuclear to cytoplasmic ratio (N/C) ratio, nucleomegaly, anisonucleosis, hyperchromasia, and irregular nuclear borders, were likewise associated with the detection of genetic alterations, giving the overall cytologic impression of a sensitivity of 27% and a specificity of 100% for NGS positivity.[29] These correlations support the continued

Table 1
Sensitivity and Specificty of Molecular Analysis of Bile Duct Brushing Specimens Compared to Cytomorphology

	Sensitivity	Specificity	Reference
Cytomorphology	0.48	0.99	Singhiet et al.,[11] 2020
	0.67	0.98	Dudleyet et al.,[10] 2016
	0.41	1.00	Kushniret et al.,[60] 2019
FISH	NA	NA	Singhi et al.,[11] 2020
	0.55	0.94	Dudley et al.,[10] 2016
	0.39	1.00	Kushnir et al.,[60] 2019
Molecular analysis	0.73	1.00	Singhi et al.,[11] 2020
	0.74	0.98	Dudley et al.,[10] 2016
	0.50	0.97	Kushnir et al.,[60] 2019
Cytomorphology + Molecular analysis	0.83	0.99	Singhi et al.,[11] 2020
	0.85	0.96	Dudley et al.,[10] 2016
	0.63	0.97	Kushnir et al.,[60] 2019
Cytomorphology + FISH + Molecular analysis	NA	NA	Singhi et al.,[11] 2020
	0.85	0.90	Dudley et al.,[10] 2016
	0.69	0.97	Kushnir et al.,[60] 2019

In Singhi et al., the molecular analysis consists of a 28 gene NGS panel (BiliSeq). In Dudley et al., the molecular analysis consists of anchored multiplex PCR targeting hotspots and exons from 39 genes. In Kushnir et al., the molecular analysis consists of a targeted PCR panel, including KRAS point mutations and tumor-suppressor gene loss of heterozygosity mutations at 10 loci. In all three studies, specimens were considered cytomorphologically positive if they were classified as either suspicious for malignancy or malignant.

value of the traditional cytomorphologic evaluation and the collection of molecular data.

OTHER METHODOLOGIES

Digital image-assisted nuclear analysis, a method of analyzing DNA content and distribution within the nucleus, has been proposed as a method for increasing the diagnostic sensitivity of biliary cytology specimens for malignant pancreaticobiliary tract strictures. Given that these methods are morphology-based, it is not surprising that the reported sensitivity and specificity are similar to cytomorphology alone, as reported by an experienced pathologist.[15] While promising, digital image analysis has shown limited uptake and is not yet recommended for diagnostic purposes. Artificial intelligence has been successfully applied to ERCP cannulation[53] and radiologic evaluation of biliary strictures;[54] however, artificial intelligence/computer-aided analysis of cytologic specimens has not yet been reported in this context.

Several noninvasive molecular methods have been suggested to differentiate CCA from benign causes of biliary stricture. These include proteometric analysis of bile and urine specimens,[55,56] detection of circulating cell-free DNA,[57] and analysis of serum microRNAs.[58,59] Although these noninvasive methods require further study, they are especially promising in that they may provide increased diagnostic sensitivity and specificity while avoiding unnecessary ERCP procedures and their associated morbidity.

SUMMARY

The continued surveillance of patients with biliary strictures using brushing cytology is undoubtedly valuable, given the challenges inherent in sampling them otherwise. Adding mutational data to cytomorphology provide a strong diagnostic benefit with increased sensitivity for the detection of biliary malignancies, which has the potential to decrease the time to a definitive diagnosis and benefit subsequent treatment planning. Within relevant publications to date, the addition of mutational data to the cytologic evaluation of BDB specimens consistently increase the sensitivity of detecting malignancy, with only modest decreases in specificity (**Table 1**).[10,60] Overall, the greatest gains in sensitivity were noted in patients with PSC, highlighting the added value of ancillary molecular analysis whereby cytomorphology is most challenging.[11,12] It is likely that molecular analysis will enter the standard of care in the diagnosis of new biliary strictures as molecular data also provide the clinical care team with prognostic information, connect patients with targeted therapies, and identify the early signs of treatment resistance.

CLINICS CARE POINTS

- Molecular analysis of biliary brushing specimens improves detection of high-risk strictures compared with cytology alone.

- Next-generation sequencing + cytology is as good as fluorescence in-situ hybridization + cytology for the early detection of malignancy.

- Molecular data provide the clinical care team with prognostic information, connect patients with targeted therapies, and identify early signs of treatment resistance.

- Rapid on-site evaluation, which requires direct smears, adds no value to bile duct brushing procedures.

- Liquid-based cytology of bile duct brushing samples provides tissue for cytology and ancillary molecular testing.

DISCLOSURE

The authors have nothing to disclose.

REFERENCES

1. Dumonceau JM, Delhaye M, Charette N, et al. Challenging biliary strictures: pathophysiological features, differential diagnosis, diagnostic algorithms, and new clinically relevant biomarkers - part 1. TherapAdvGastroenterol 2020;13:1–27.

2. Yin SM, Liu YW, Liu YY, et al. Short-term outcomes after minimally invasive versus open pancreaticoduodenectomy in elderly patients: a propensity score-matched analysis. BMCSurg 2021;21(1):60.

3. Cambridge WA, Fairfield C, Powell JJ, et al. Meta-analysis and Meta-regression of Survival After Liver Transplantation for UnresectablePerihilarCholangiocarcinoma. Ann Surg 2021;273(2):240–50.

4. Sardar M, Shroff RT. Biliary Cancer: Gateway to comprehensive molecular profiling. ClinAdvHematolOncol 2021;19(1):27–34.

5. Tummala P, Munigala S, Eloubeidi MA, et al. Patients With Obstructive Jaundice and Biliary Stricture±Mass Lesion on Imaging. Prevalence of Malignancy and Potential Role of EUS-FNA. J ClinGastroenterol 2013;47(6):532–7.

6. Singh A, Gelrud A, Agarwal B. Biliary strictures: diagnostic considerations and approach. Gastroenterol Rep (Oxf) 2015;3(1):22–31.

7. Barr Fritcher EG, Kipp BR, Slezak JM, et al. Correlating routine cytology, quantitative nuclear morphometry by digital image analysis, and genetic alterations by fluorescence in situ hybridization to assess the sensitivity of cytology for detecting pancreatobiliary tract malignancy. Am J ClinPathol 2007;128(2):272–9.

8. Govil H, Reddy V, Kluskens L, et al. Brush cytology of the biliary tract: retrospective study of 278 cases with histopathologic correlation. DiagnCytopathol 2002;26(5):273–7.

9. Kipp BR, Stadheim LM, Halling SA, et al. A comparison of routine cytology and fluorescence in situ hybridization for the detection of malignant bile duct strictures. Am J Gastroenterol 2004;99(9):1675–81.

10. Dudley JC, Zheng Z, McDonald T, et al. Next-Generation Sequencing and Fluorescence in Situ Hybridization Have Comparable Performance Characteristics in the Analysis of Pancreaticobiliary Brushings for Malignancy. J MolDiagn 2016;18(1):124–30.

11. Singhi AD, Nikiforova MN, Chennat J, et al. Integrating next-generation sequencing to endoscopic retrograde cholangiopancreatography (ERCP)-obtained biliary specimens improves the detection and management of patients with malignant bile duct strictures. Gut 2020;69(1):52–61.

12. Scheid JF, Rosenbaum MW, Przybyszewski EM, et al. Next-generation sequencing in the evaluation of biliary strictures in patients with primary sclerosing cholangitis. Cancer Cytopathol 2022;130(3):215–30. https://doi.org/10.1002/cncy.22528. Epub 2021 Nov 2. PMID: 34726838.

13. de Bellis M, Sherman S, Fogel EL, et al. Tissue sampling at ERCP in suspected malignant biliary strictures (Part 2). GastrointestEndosc 2002;56(5):720–30.

14. Yamaguchi T, Shirai Y, Nakamura N, et al. Usefulness of Brush Cytology Combined With Pancreatic Juice Cytology in the Diagnosis of Pancreatic Cancer. Pancreas 2012;41(8):1225–9.

15. Uehara H, Tatsumi K, Masuda E, et al. Scraping cytology with a guidewire for pancreatic-ductal strictures. GastrointestEndosc 2009;70(1):52–9.

16. Kamp E, Dinjens WNM, Doukas M, et al. Optimal tissue sampling during ERCP and emerging molecular techniques for the differentiation of benign and malignant biliary strictures. TherapAdvGastroenterol 2021;14:1–24.

17. Polkowski M, Jenssen C, Kaye P, et al. Technical aspects of endoscopic ultrasound (EUS)-guided sampling in gastroenterology: European Society of Gastrointestinal Endoscopy (ESGE) Technical Guideline - March 2017. Endoscopy 2017;49(10):989–1006.

18. Pitman MB, Layfield LJ. Guidelines for pancreaticobiliary cytology from the Papanicolaou Society of Cytopathology: A review. Cancer Cytopathol 2014;122(6):399–411.

19. Navaneethan U, Njei B, Lourdusamy V, et al. Comparative effectiveness of biliary brush cytology

and intraductal biopsy for detection of malignant biliary strictures: a systematic review and meta-analysis. GastrointestEndosc 2015;81(1):168–76.

20. Onoyama T, Takeda Y, Kawata S, et al. Adequate tissue acquisition rate of peroralcholangioscopy-guided forceps biopsy. Ann Transl Med 2020;8(17):1073.

21. Baron TH. Endoscopic retrograde cholangiopancreatography for cholangiocarcinoma. ClinLiver Dis 2014;18(4):891–7.

22. Novikov A, Kowalski TE, Loren DE. Practical Management of Indeterminate Biliary Strictures. GastrointestEndoscClin N Am 2019;29(2):205–14.

23. Cohen MB, Wittchow RJ, Johlin FC, et al. Brush cytology of the extrahepatic biliary tract: comparison of cytologic features of adenocarcinoma and benign biliary strictures. Mod Pathol 1995;8(5):498–502.

24. Layfield LJ, Wax TD, Lee JG, et al. Accuracy and morphologic aspects of pancreatic and biliary duct brushings. ActaCytol 1995;39(1):11–8.

25. Nakajima T, Tajima Y, Sugano I, et al. Multivariate statistical analysis of bile cytology. ActaCytol 1994; 38(1):51–5.

26. Xu X, Kobayashi S, Qiao W, et al. Induction of intrahepatic cholangiocellular carcinoma by liver-specific disruption of Smad4 and Pten in mice. J Clin Invest 2006;116(7):1843–52.

27. Volmar KE, Vollmer RT, Routbort MJ, et al. Pancreatic and bile duct brushing cytology in 1000 cases: review of findings and comparison of preparation methods. Cancer 2006;108(4):231–8.

28. Salomao M, Gonda TA, Margolskee E, et al. Strategies for improving diagnostic accuracy of biliary strictures. Cancer Cytopathol 2015;123(4):244–52.

29. Rosenbaum MW, Arpin R, Limbocker J, et al. Cytomorphologic characteristics of next-generation sequencing-positive bile duct brushing specimens. J Am SocCytopathol 2020;9(6):520–7.

30. Barr Fritcher EG, Caudill JL, Blue JE, et al. Identification of malignant cytologic criteria in pancreatobiliary brushings with corresponding positive fluorescence in situ hybridization results. Am J ClinPathol 2011;136(3):442–9.

31. Renshaw AA, Madge R, Jiroutek M, et al. Bile duct brushing cytology: statistical analysis of proposed diagnostic criteria. Am J ClinPathol 1998;110(5):635–40.

32. Kitajima Y, Ohara H, Nakazawa T, et al. Usefulness of transpapillary bile duct brushing cytology and forceps biopsy for improved diagnosis in patients with biliary strictures. J GastroenterolHepatol 2007; 22(10):1615–20.

33. Naitoh I, Nakazawa T, Kato A, et al. Predictive factors for positive diagnosis of malignant biliary strictures by transpapillarybrush cytology and forceps biopsy. J Dig Dis 2016;17(1):44–51.

34. Chadwick BE, Layfield LJ, Witt BL, et al. Significance of atypia in pancreatic and bile duct brushings: follow-up analysis of the categories atypical

and suspicious for malignancy. DiagnCytopathol 2014;42(4):285–91.

35. Hoda RS, Finer EB, Arpin RN 3rd, et al. Risk of malignancy in the categories of the Papanicolaou Society of Cytopathology system for reporting pancreaticobiliary cytology. J Am SocCytopathol 2019;8(3):120–7.

36. Pitman MB, Layfield L. The Papanicolaou Society of Cytopathology System for reporting pancreaticobiliary cytology. 1st edition. Switzerland: Springer International Publishing; 2015.

37. Vandervoort J, Soetikno RM, Montes H, et al. Accuracy and complication rate of brush cytology from bile duct versus pancreatic duct. GastrointestEndosc 1999;49(3 Pt 1):322–7.

38. Yeo MK, Kim KH, Lee YM, et al. The usefulness of adding p53 immunocytochemistry to bile drainage cytology for the diagnosis of malignant biliary strictures. DiagnCytopathol 2017;45(7):592–7.

39. Moreno Luna LE, Kipp B, Halling KC, et al. Advanced Cytologic Techniques for the Detection of Malignant Pancreatobiliary Strictures. Gastroenterology 2006;131(4):1064–72.

40. Barr Fritcher EG, Voss JS, Jenkins SM, et al. Primary sclerosing cholangitis with equivocal cytology: fluorescence in situ hybridization and serum CA 19-9 predict risk of malignancy. Cancer Cytopathol 2013;121(12):708–17.

41. Barr Fritcher EG, Kipp BR, Voss JS, et al. Primary sclerosing cholangitis patients with serial polysomy fluorescence in situ hybridization results are at increased risk of cholangiocarcinoma. Am J Gastroenterol 2011;106(11):2023–8.

42. Kerr SE, Barr Fritcher EG, Campion MB, et al. Biliary dysplasia in primary sclerosing cholangitis harbors cytogenetic abnormalities similar to cholangiocarcinoma. Hum Pathol 2014;45(9):1797–804.

43. Rizvi S, Eaton J, Yang JD, et al. Emerging Technologies for the Diagnosis of PerihilarCholangiocarcinoma. SeminLiver Dis 2018;38(2):160–9.

44. Bergquist ATB, Glaumann H, Broome U. Can DNA cytometry be used for evaluation of malignanty and premalignancy in bile duct strictures in Primary Sclerosing Cholangitis? J Hepatol 2000;33:873–7.

45. Wardell CP, Fujita M, Yamada T, et al. Genomic characterization of biliary tract cancers identifies driver genes and predisposing mutations. J Hepatol 2018;68(5):959–69.

46. Razumilava N, Gores GJ. Cholangiocarcinoma. Lancet 2014;383(9935):2168–79.

47. Chung JY, Hong SM, Choi BY, et al. The expression of phospho-AKT, phospho-mTOR, and PTEN in extrahepaticcholangiocarcinoma. ClinCancer Res 2009;15(2):660–7.

48. Jain A, Borad MJ, Kelley RK, et al. Cholangiocarcinoma with FGFR genetic aberrations: A unique clinical phenotype. JCO Precision Oncol 2018;2:1–12.

49. Maruki Y, Morizane C, Arai Y, et al. Molecular detection and clinicopathological characteristics of advanced/recurrent biliary tract carcinomas harboring the FGFR2 rearrangements: a prospective observational study (PRELUDE Study). J Gastroenterol 2021;56(3):250–60.

50. Javle M, Bekaii-Saab T, Jain A, et al. Biliary cancer: Utility of next-generation sequencing for clinical management. Cancer 2016;122(24):3838–47.

51. O'Rourke CJ, Munoz-Garrido P, Andersen JB. Molecular Targets in Cholangiocarcinoma. Hepatology 2021;73(Suppl 1):62–74.

52. Abou-Alfa GK, Sahai V, Hollebecque A, et al. Pemigatinib for previously treated, locally advanced or metastatic cholangiocarcinoma: a multicentre, open-label, phase 2 study. LancetOncol 2020; 21(5):671–84.

53. Kim T, Kim J, Choi HS, et al. Artificial intelligence-assisted analysis of endoscopic retrograde cholangiopancreatography image for identifying ampulla and difficulty of selective cannulation. Scientific Rep 2021;11(8381). https://doi.org/10.1038/s41598-021-87737-3.

54. Yang CM, Shu J. Cholangiocarcinoma Evaluation via Imaging and Artificial Intelligence. Oncology 2021; 99:72–83.

55. Lankisch TO, Metzger J, Negm AA, et al. Bile proteomic profiles differentiate cholangiocarcinoma from primary sclerosing cholangitis and choledocholithiasis. Hepatology 2011;53(3):875–84.

56. Metzger J, Negm AA, Plentz RR, et al. Urine proteomic analysis differentiates cholangiocarcinoma from primary sclerosing cholangitis and other benign biliary disorders. Gut 2013;62(1):122–30.

57. Zill OA, Greene C, Sebisanovic D, et al. Cell-Free DNA Next-Generation Sequencing in Pancreatobiliary Carcinomas. CancerDiscov 2015;5(10):1040–8.

58. Bernuzzi F, Marabita F, Lleo A, et al. Serum microRNAs as novel biomarkers for primary sclerosing cholangitis and cholangiocarcinoma. ClinExpImmunol 2016;185(1):61–71.

59. Le N, Fillinger J, Szanyi S, et al. Analysis of microRNA expression in brush cytology specimens improves the diagnosis of pancreatobiliary cancer. Pancreatology 2019;19:873–9.

60. Kushnir VM, Mullady DK, Das K, et al. The Diagnostic Yield of Malignancy Comparing Cytology, FISH, and Molecular Analysis of Cell Free Cytology Brush Supernatant in Patients With Biliary Strictures Undergoing Endoscopic Retrograde Cholangiography (ERC): A Prospective Study. J ClinGastroenterol 2019;53(9):686–92.

Advances in the Surgical Treatment of Pancreatic Cancer

Jian Zheng, MD, Alessandro Paniccia, MD,
Amer H. Zureikat, MD*

KEYWORDS

• Minimally invasive pancreatectomy • Neoadjuvant therapy • Irreversible electroporation

---

Key points

- Minimally invasive distal pancreatectomy is associated with improved or comparable perioperative outcomes compared with open surgery, although more evidence is needed to establish benefits for minimally invasive pancreaticoduodenectomy.

- Neoadjuvant therapy leads to increased R0 resection rates and sterilization of regional lymph nodes and allows in vivo assessment of tumor response. It is considered the standard of care for borderline resectable or locally advanced pancreatic cancer, but its advantages in resectable cancer remain to be demonstrated.

- Irreversible electroporation may offer survival benefits for patients with locally advanced pancreatic cancer, but future prospective randomized controlled trials are needed to validate its merits over current modern chemotherapy.

ABSTRACT

Three recent advances in the surgical approach to pancreatic cancer over the past decade have improved both short- and long-term outcomes for patients with nonmetastatic, operable pancreatic cancer. These include (1) minimally invasive pancreatectomy to reduce operative morbidity while adhering to principles of open oncologic resections, (2) neoadjuvant chemotherapy to treat radiographically occult metastatic disease and improve locoregional control, and (3) applying irreversible electroporation as an adjunct to surgery, allowing a fraction of locally advanced pancreatic cancer to be resected.

OVERVIEW

Pancreatic ductal adenocarcinoma (PDAC) is the fourth leading cause of cancer-related death in the United States.[1] Performing an oncologic resection with microscopic negative margins and regional lymphadenectomy offers the best chance for cure, but less than 20% of patients are diagnosed with operable cancer at presentation.[1,2] Although the overall 5-year survival is only 9% because of the high incidence of metastatic disease at presentation, this can be improved to approximately 30% for resected patients in the setting of multimodality therapy.[3] It is thus imperative to couple curative intent resection with multidisciplinary treatments including systemic and regional therapies to prolong both recurrence-free and overall survival.[4,5]

Three recent advances in the surgical treatment of PDAC have improved both perioperative and long-term outcomes. First, minimally invasive pancreatectomy, although slow to adopt due to technical challenges, has led to improved perioperative outcomes without compromising oncologic outcomes. This is particularly true for distal pancreatectomy, although more evidence is

---

Division of Surgical Oncology, University of Pittsburgh Medical Center, 5150 Centre Avenue, Suite 421, UPMC Cancer Pavilion, Pittsburgh, PA 15232, USA
* Corresponding author.
E-mail address: zureikatah@upmc.edu

Surgical Pathology 15 (2022) 479–490
https://doi.org/10.1016/j.path.2022.05.003
1875-9181/22/© 2022 Elsevier Inc. All rights reserved.

needed for minimally invasive pancreaticoduodenectomy (PD). Second, neoadjuvant chemotherapy with or without radiation has led to increased rates of R0 resection, decreased regional lymph node positivity, and prolonged survival in patients with borderline (BR) and locally advanced (LA) PDAC, although the benefits remain less clear for resectable PDAC. Third, the use of locoregional therapy with irreversible electroporation (IRE) may offer survival benefits for patients with LA-PDAC, but more trials are needed to validate this modality over modern-day effective chemotherapy. This article discusses these advances in detail.

MINIMALLY INVASIVE PANCREATECTOMY

Since the first introduction of minimally invasive surgery (MIS) for pancreatic tumors in the early 1990s, its adoption has been approached with cautious optimism because of operative complexity, postoperative morbidity, and concerns for oncologic efficacy.[6] Despite this slow adoption, MIS approaches—which include laparoscopic and robotic techniques—are now increasingly performed and have even become standard practice in many high-volume centers with experienced MIS surgeons.[6]

From a surgical perspective, improved long-term survival following pancreatic resection depends on several prognostic factors that include negative resection margins and adequate regional lymph node dissection for accurate staging.[2,7] In addition, lower operative blood loss and transfusion rates are associated with improved recurrence-free and overall survival, likely related to the immunosuppressive effect of blood products on cancer cells as they escape immunologic detection and disseminate.[8] Although the surgical approaches do not alter the biology of PDAC, a sound surgical technique that results in fewer complications and minimizes the decline in performance status allows for earlier administration of systemic adjuvant therapy.

In the hands of experienced surgeons, margin negative resections and lymph node harvest are comparable in minimally invasive and open pancreatectomy, with some studies indicating higher lymph node yield for robotic pancreatectomy compared with the open approach.[9] A critical step in achieving margin negative resections and adequate lymph node sampling is meticulous dissection of the retroperitoneal margin during PD. Even in the setting of BR-PDAC, in which a short segment of superior mesenteric or portal vein abutment is encountered, both robotic and laparoscopic approaches can be safely used to perform

lateral venorrhaphy with vascular endostapler (**Fig. 1**) or hand-sewn technique (or even rarely end-to-end anastomosis) to obtain negative margin at the vascular groove.[10] This was demonstrated in two large series from the University of Pittsburgh (robotic) and Mayo Clinic (laparoscopic).[10,11] The authors have adopted the robotic platform as the favored approach for minimally invasive pancreatic resection because of several advantages over standard laparoscopy including 3D visualization, magnification, enhanced dexterity, precision, and favorable ergonomics. Several single, multi-institutional, and national series have now confirmed that the robotic approach is associated with fewer conversions and potentially less complications compared with laparoscopy, particularly for PD.[12–14]

For PD, four randomized controlled trials have been reported comparing minimally invasive and open PD for periampullary pathology (**Table 1**).[15–19] Both the PLOT and PADULAP trials recruited patients from India and Spain, respectively, and demonstrated shorter length of stay for laparoscopic PD, while achieving comparable oncologic outcomes (including the number of lymph nodes retrieved and rates of margin negative resection), and postoperative complication rates as stratified by Clavien–Dindo grades and clinically relevant postoperative pancreatic fistula (CR-POPF) rates.[15,16] A third trial, LEOPARD-2 trial from the Netherlands, was terminated prematurely because of safety concerns over the increased 90-day mortality in the laparoscopic PD cohort.[17,18] A more recent large multicenter trial from China randomized more than 600 patients to laparoscopic versus open PD and confirmed a shorter length of stay (1 day) for laparoscopic PD with all other outcomes being comparable.[19] Limitations of these trials include their lack of inclusion of robotic PD and their inclusion of heterogenous periampullary pathology.

Importantly, for robotic PD, no randomized controlled trials have been performed comparing this platform to open or laparoscopic PD. These trials are difficult to conduct because even in high-volume centers, loosely defined as 20 cases per year, and even with robust robotic training programs, approximately 80 cases are needed to optimize the learning curve as shown by the authors' analysis of their robotic PD learning curve. In this analysis of their first 200 robotic pancreatoduodenectomy (RPDs), improvements in the rates of conversion to open and operative blood loss occurred after 20 cases (35.0% vs 3.3% [*P* < .001], and 600 mL vs 250 mL [*P* = .002], respectively), whereas reduction in clinically relevant postoperative pancreatic fistula occurred

Fig. 1. Robotic lateral venorrhaphy using vascular endostapler for portal vein tumor abutment.

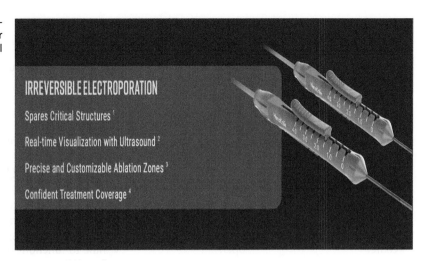

after 40 cases (27.5% vs 14.4%; *P* = .04) and improvements in operating room time after 80 cases (581 vs 417 min [*P* < .001]).[20,21] Although ongoing trials are accruing, the best current evidence on the safety and feasibility of robotic PD is a study of eight high-volume pancreatic centers in the United States, comparing open PD (*N* = 817) and robotic PD (*N* = 211).[22] In this analysis, robotic PD was associated with lower operative blood loss, longer operative time, and lower rates of major complications.[22] In the sub-analysis of patients with PDAC, robotic PD was associated with comparable rates of R0 resection and adequate nodal harvest ($\geq$12 lymph nodes) to open PD.[22] In an another study from the National Cancer Database, patients with stage 1 to 3 PDAC who underwent robotic PD (*N* = 626) had a similar median overall survival of approximately 22 months as compared with those who underwent an open operation (*N* = 17,205).[23]

For distal pancreatectomy (DP), randomized controlled trials more clearly indicate benefits to

Table 1
Randomized controlled trials comparing laparoscopic and open pancreaticoduodenectomy[15–19]

Trials	Trial Details	Laparoscopic vs Open Pancreaticoduodenectomy Results
PLOT (India, 2017)[15] Single center	*N* = 32 lap vs *N* = 32 open	• Operative blood loss (median 250 vs 401 mL, *P*<.001) • Operative time (median 359 vs 320 min, *P* = .041) • Length of stay (median 7 vs 13 d, *P* = .001) • Comparable lymph node yield, R0 resection, CR-POPF, delayed gastric emptying, post-pancreatectomy hemorrhage, Clavien–Dindo grade $\geq$ 3, and 90-d mortality
PADULAP (Spain, 2018)[16] Single center	*N* = 32 lap vs *N* = 29 open	• Operative time (median 486 vs 365 min, *P* = .0001) • Length of stay (median 13.5 vs 15 d, *P* = .024) • Clavien–Dindo grade $\geq$ 3 (*N* = 5 vs *N* = 11, *P* = .040) • Comprehensive complication index score (20.6 vs 29.6, *P* = .038) • Poor quality outcome (*N* = 10 vs *N* = 14, *P* = .041) • Comparable lymph node yield, R0 margin, transfusion requirement, and pancreas-specific complications
LEOPARD-2 (the Netherlands, 2019)[17,18] 4 centers	*N* = 50 lap vs *N* = 49 open	• Closed prematurely because of the 90-d complication-related mortality in *N* = 5 (10%) after laparoscopic vs *N* = 1 (2%) after open pancreaticoduodenectomy • Comparable time to functional recovery, Clavien–Dindo grade $\geq$ 3, and CR-POPF
MITG-P-CPAM trial (China, 2021)[19] 14 centers	*N* = 328 lap vs *N* = 328 open	• Length of stay (median 15 vs 16 d, *P* = .020) • Comparable 90-d mortality, Clavien–Dindo grade $\geq$ 3, and comprehensive complication index score

Table 2
Randomized controlled trials comparing laparoscopic and open distal pancreatectomy[24,25]

Trials	Trial Details	MIS vs Open DP Results
LEOPARD (Netherlands, 2019)[24] 14 centers	N = 51 MIS vs N = 57 open	• Operative blood loss (150 vs 400 mL, P<.001) • Operative time (217 vs 179 min, P = .005) • Time to functional recovery (4 vs 6 d, P<.001) • Delayed gastric emptying grade B/C (6% vs 20%, P = .04) • Quality of life (days 3–30) was significantly better after MIS DP compared with open DP (P = .003) • Comparable CR-POPF, Clavien–Dindo grade ≥ 3, and 90-d mortality
LAPOP (Sweden, 2020)[25] 1 center	N = 29 MIS vs N = 29 open	• Operative blood loss (50 < 100 mL, P = .018) • Time to functional recovery (4 vs 6 d, P = .007) • Length of stay (5 vs 6 d, P = .002) • Comparable operative time, CR-POPF, Clavien–Dindo grade ≥ 3, delayed gastric emptying, and post-pancreatectomy hemorrhage

MIS over open surgery (**Table 2**).[24,25] The LEOPARD trial from the Netherlands randomized 108 patients to open or MIS DP including laparoscopic and robotic approaches. MIS was associated with less operative blood loss, reduced delayed gastric emptying, shorter time to functional recovery, and improved quality of life scores.[24] There were no differences in Clavien–Dindo grade 3 complications, CR-POPF, or 90-day mortality.[24] Similar advantages for MID DP were also concluded in the LAPOP trial from Sweden.[25]

In summary, minimally invasive pancreatectomy for pancreatic cancer is being increasingly performed by surgeons with MIS expertise. In highly selected patients, improvements in outcomes can be achieved especially if performed at high-volume centers. MIS distal pancreatectomy has been associated with improved perioperative outcomes compared with the open approach, although more evidence is needed to demonstrate meaningful benefits for MIS PD. Based on the increasing utilization of minimally invasive approaches to pancreatectomy, the Miami International Evidence-Based Guidelines in 2019 were formulated to standardize the practice of minimally invasive pancreatectomy while at the same time proposing actions to further advance this field.[21]

NEOADJUVANT THERAPY

Although surgery is the only hope for a potential cure, systemic therapy is an important component of the multimodality care in operable PDAC.

Adjuvant therapy is now the standard of care following resection based on several randomized trials using single-agent gemcitabine or 5FU.[3,26,27] These single-agent regimens, however, are associated with a modest survival advantage because of their low response rates of 8% to 12%. The last decade has witnessed the incorporation of more effective multidrug adjuvant regimens such as FOLFIRINOX (folic acid, fluorouracil, irinotecan, and oxaliplatin) and gemcitabine with nab-paclitaxel or capecitabine in the adjuvant setting because of their higher response rates and improved survival rates compared with monotherapy alone.[4,5,28] Owing to the morbidity of pancreatic resections, however, only 50% of the patients are able to initiate and complete adjuvant therapy, making upfront systemic therapy a prudent strategy.[29] In particular, neoadjuvant FOLFIRINOX or gemcitabine/nab-paclitaxel is now the standard of care in BR-PDAC, although a clear survival benefit over adjuvant therapy remains to be firmly demonstrated in randomized trials when evaluating for both resectable and BR-PDAC.[30,31] Moreover, the nature of the neoadjuvant regimen, its duration, and the added value of radiation in this setting remain to be established. Thus, patient treatment plans should be determined by multidisciplinary tumor boards that take into consideration several aspects of pancreatic cancer care including anatomic resectability criteria, biological factors such as cancer (CA) 19-9 levels, and patient performance status. Below are the putative advantages of neoadjuvant therapy over a surgery-first approach in patients with PDAC:

1. *Downsizing PDAC increases margin negative resection and sterilizes regional LN.* Approximately 30% of patients with PDAC present with BR or LA PDAC due to involvement of regional vasculature. Such anatomic criteria of resectability are clearly defined by the NCCN.[29] In the context of BR and LA-PDAC, such resections are likely to be associated with positive margins if treated with upfront surgery. Although neoadjuvant therapy may not downstage tumors radiographically, it allows for increased rates of R0 resection when compared with a surgery-first approach, with or without vascular resection and reconstruction.[29,30]

   - Several early trials from MD Anderson laid the foundation for neoadjuvant therapy nearly 2 decades ago.[32–34] In a phase II trial, 86 patients with potentially resectable stage I or II PDAC received neoadjuvant gemcitabine-based chemoradiation.[32] In total, 74% underwent a successful PD after neoadjuvant therapy, of which 90% achieved an R0 resection and 62% were N0.[32] The median survival was 34 months for those who underwent PD compared with only 7 months for unresected patients (*P*<.001).[32] In the same study, histologic assessment of treatment effect on the resected specimen revealed that using gemcitabine as the radiosensitizer generated greater tumor cell kill than using 5-FU or paclitaxel administered in prior studies.[32–34]
   - In a multicenter randomized controlled trial (NCT01458717) from four high-volume centers in Korea, 27 patients with BR-PDAC were assigned to gemcitabine-based neoadjuvant chemoradiation therapy followed by surgery versus 23 patients who were randomized to upfront surgery.[35] The neoadjuvant cohort achieved a significantly higher rate of R0 resection compared with upfront surgery (51.8% vs 26.1%, *P* = .004), providing additional support for neoadjuvant therapy.[35] Although not powered for survival differences, patients who received neoadjuvant chemoradiation had significantly improved 2-year and median overall survival compared with upfront surgery (40.7%, 21 months vs 26.1%, 12 months, respectively, *P* = .028).[35]
   - Consideration is now being given to a total neoadjuvant therapy strategy for patients with BR-PDAC to maximize R0 resection rates. Of the 48 patients who were enrolled in a phase II clinical trials with 8 weeks of neoadjuvant FOLFIRINOX followed by neoadjuvant chemoradiation, 31 (65%) patients had R0 resection.[36] The median overall survival was 37.7 months among all enrolled patients. It remains unclear if these remarkable results are attributed to the greater number of cycles received preoperatively or a direct function of improved patient selection offered by the prolonged preoperative period of observation.
   - For LA-PDAC, the median survival averages 9 to 11 months, and less than 20% of patients typically can be ultimately resected.[37] The use of modified FOLFIRINOX with or without radiation for LA-PDAC was evaluated in a prospective study from 11 French centers.[37] Of the 77 patients enrolled, 28 (36%) patients underwent a resection with 24 (86%) achieving R0 resection.[37] Although only a minority of patients ultimately underwent resection, those resected achieved a median overall survival of 22 months.[37] A large meta-analysis of 11 studies representing 315 patients with LA-PDAC following FOLFIRINOX treatment revealed median overall survival of 24.2 months and median progression-free survival of 15.0 months.[38] The random effects model revealed that 25.9% proceeded to get curative-intent resection, among which 74.1% of patients had an R0 resection.[38]
   - Although many centers are adopting a neoadjuvant approach, no survival benefit has yet to be proven in a randomized trial study design, especially for resectable PDAC. Although we await the results of the Alliance A021806 trial, which examines a strategy of neoadjuvant FOLFIRINOX versus upfront surgery followed by adjuvant FOLFIRINOX, other recent trials have demonstrated some interesting results.[29] The PREOPANC trial was a randomized phase III study of 16 Dutch centers, which randomized patients with resectable or BR-PDAC to neoadjuvant chemoradiotherapy versus immediate pancreatectomy.[31] In this study, the median overall survival by intention to treat was not significantly different between the two arms (16 vs 14.3 months, *P* = .096).[31] However, those who received neoadjuvant chemoradiation did achieve a higher rate of R0 resection at 71% compared with 40% of those assigned to immediate surgery (*P*<.001) and were associated with significantly better disease-free survival.[31] In the subgroup analysis,

those with resectable PDAC did not achieve a survival benefit with neoadjuvant therapy, whereas those with BR-PDAC did. Thus, more prospective studies are needed to better clarify the value of neoadjuvant therapy for patients with resectable PDAC.

- In SWOG S1505, the safety and efficacy of perioperative (3 months of neoadjuvant and 3 months of adjuvant) FOLFIRINOX and gemcitabine/nab-paclitaxel for resectable PDAC were compared.[28] This study demonstrated that of 103 eligible patients, 77 (76%) completed neoadjuvant therapy and underwent surgery.[28] Among the 73 patients successfully resected, 62 (85%) had R0 resection, 31 (42%) were N0, and 24 (33%) had a complete or major pathologic response to neoadjuvant therapy.[28] Although this trial demonstrated a lack of superiority of one regimen over the other, the median survival was disappointingly low at 23 months on an intent to treat basis.[39] This analysis, in our assessment, highlights the need for a precision-based approach to neoadjuvant therapy in operable pancreatic cancer. It is likely that subsets of tumors respond preferentially to gemcitabine-based or 5-FU-based regimens, but not both. Identifying these subsets of patients will likely realize the full benefits of neoadjuvant therapy.

2. *Neoadjuvant therapy increases the likelihood of completing chemotherapy cycles.* A significant proportion of patients do not receive their intended adjuvant therapy following pancreatectomy due to postoperative complications, worsening performance status, and early cancer progression.[40,41]

    - In a study from MD Anderson, multimodality therapy completion rates were evaluated among patients with resectable PDAC treated either with neoadjuvant therapy first or with surgery-first approaches.[41] The authors reported that 83% of patients treated with a neoadjuvant approach ultimately completed multimodality therapy, compared with only 58% who had surgery-first approach.[41] Patients who completed multimodality therapy had a median overall survival that was over three times longer (36 vs 11 months, $P<.001$).[41] The most common reason for failure to complete multimodality therapy was early disease progression, which occurred at a rate of 11% in the neoadjuvant group versus 26% in the surgery-first group, whereas major postoperative major complication rates were similar between both groups.[41]

However, among patients who underwent surgery-first approach, 69% with no major complication completed multimodality therapies, compared to 29% with major complications ($P = .040$).[41] Thus, the authors concluded that neoadjuvant therapy offered a practical clinical advantage, especially for patients with poor biology and high operative risks.

- In a larger study of 2047 patients with data obtained from the American College of Surgeons National Surgical Quality Improvement Program and the National Cancer Database, only 57.7% of patients with stage 1 or 2 PDAC received adjuvant chemotherapy after resection.[42] Approximately 23.2% of patients in this study developed at least one serious complication postoperatively, which doubled the likelihood of not receiving any adjuvant therapy and the likelihood of delaying adjuvant therapy by $\geq$ 70 days.[42]
- A more recent National Cancer Database analysis suggested that despite advances in surgical care, the rate of omission of chemotherapy remained unchanged during the study period (2006–2016).[43] This finding emphasized the inherent delayed recovery associated with pancreatectomy. In this study, patients who failed to receive adjuvant chemotherapy but were treated with neoadjuvant chemotherapy had a similar survival to those who received planned adjuvant chemotherapy (26.9 vs 24.7 months, $P = .21$).[43] The authors suggested that the use of chemotherapy in the preoperative period may lessen the deleterious survival impact of omission of adjuvant chemotherapy. Collectively, the delivery of neoadjuvant chemotherapy increases the likelihood that patients complete their intended systemic therapy.

3. *Neoadjuvant therapy can identify pateints with aggressive tumor biology, select patients who would benefit from surgery, and help guide adjuvant therapy.* One of the undeniable benefits of neoadjuvant therapy is that it allows for careful assessment of tumor biology. Indeed, the biological aggressiveness of PDAC can be monitored based on (a) changing levels of CA 19-9 during neoadjuvant therapy, (b) detection of metastatic disease based on radiologic restaging during neoadjuvant therapy, and (c) by the assessment of histopathologic response to therapy in the surgical specimen which ultimately will inform the choice of adjuvant

therapy. A growing body of evidence suggests that following neoadjuvant therapy, patients who demonstrate biochemical (CA 19-9) or histopathologic features of response (CAP 0 and 1, or Evans grades III and IV) experience improved survival after resection.[44,45] On the other hand, patients who demonstrate progression during neoadjuvant therapy either radiographically or biochemically—which occurs in approximately 10% to 30%—are unlikely to derive significant benefit from resection and thus can be spared the potential morbidity of a futile operation.[44]

- In a multicenter, retrospective study, 274 patients with PDAC received neoadjuvant FOLFIRINOX or gemcitabine/nab-paclitaxel followed by pancreatectomy.[45] A marked decrease in the CA 19-9 levels by more than 50% was observed in 70% and 79% of patients, and normalization was seen in 35.9% and 35.2%, respectively.[45] Complete pathologic response was identified in 6% of patients, whereas 56.4% had a partial pathologic response, and 37.7% had no or limited pathologic response.[45] The overall, local recurrence-free, and metastasis-free survival were all significantly better in patients who had marked response in CA 19-9 levels and complete pathologic response.[45]

- The biochemical response of CA 19-9 to neoadjuvant therapy is a strong prognostic factor that may help guide plans for adjuvant therapy following resection. In a retrospective study, compared with patients with normal preoperative CA 19-9, failure to normalize preoperative or postoperative CA19-9 was associated with a 2.77-fold and 4.03-fold increase in the risk of death, respectively (P<.003).[44] According to another retrospective study, only suboptimal responders to neoadjuvant therapy (defined as no normalization of CA 19-9 and decrease of CA 19-9 in < 50%) benefitted from adjuvant therapy (overall survival 34.5 vs 19.1 months, P<.001).[46] However, in optimal responders who had normalization of CA 19-9 with decrease of more than 50% of CA 19-9 during neoadjuvant therapy, adjuvant therapy was not associated with an additional survival benefit (40.6 vs 39.0 months, P = .815).[46] These provocative data suggest that CA 19-9 therapy may guide a strategy of total neoadjuvant therapy.

- Owing to the central role of CA19-9 in gauging chemo-response, the authors obtain monthly CA19-9 levels while on NAT. These levels inform the need for continuation of the same chemotherapy regimen (in the case of CA19-9 decline), change in neoadjuvant chemotherapy regimen and/or need for radiographic restaging (CA19-9 stagnation or increase), or proceed to resection (normalization or large decline in value). The multidisciplinary care of PDAC requires a dynamic and individualized approach, coupling CA 19-9 levels with radiographic restaging to assess in vivo therapeutic response. Following resection, the NCCN recommends initiating adjuvant therapy within 12 weeks postoperatively. Pending patients' clinical and pathologic response to neoadjuvant therapy, tolerance of neoadjuvant therapy, and postoperative recovery, further adjuvant chemotherapy may be considered and tailored to the patients need with three regimens currently available for use (FOLFIRNOX, gemcitabine and capecitabine, and gemcitabine alone).[40]

- More recently, transciptomic analysis of PDAC have identified, reflecting significant tumor heterogeneity that may have significant prognostic and therapeutic relevance.[47,48] Two main tumor subtypes described are the basal-like and classical subtypes. The basal-like subtype has a worse prognosis, is characterized by epithelial-to-mesenchymal transition and TP53 expression, is often poorly differentiated, and shows poor response to 5FU chemotherapy.[47] On the other hand, the classical subtype is associated with epithelial genes and pancreatic transcription factors, has high expression of GATA6, is often well differentiated, and seems to respond better to FOLFIRINOX.[47] An increased understanding of these tumor subtypes may have implication in tailoring perioperative systemic therapy.

- In addition, to CA 19-9 and GATA6, circulating tumor cells (CTC) have been associated with a high risk of micrometastatic disease and should prompt a neoadjuvant approach even in patients with resectable disease. Coupled with other high-risk features such as large tumor size greater than 3 cm, presence of clinical (EUS, CT, or PET) nodal positivity, high CA 19-9 levels, and excessive weight loss, high levels of CTCs are prognostic and may have therapeutic implications.[40,49,50] The prospective CLUSTER study, for example, demonstrated that 96% of resectable patients had CTCs in their peripheral blood.[50] Patients who received neoadjuvant therapy had significantly lower CTCs compared with untreated patients eligible for upfront resection.[50] Although resection results in a significant reduction of CTCs, it does not eradicate them.[50] Consequently, fluctuations of CTCs may be associated with response to treatment and can precede gross recurrence as demonstrated in this study.[50]

4. *Neoadjuvant therapy is not only cytotoxic but may also help shape the cancer microenvironment.*

- In an interesting study, neoadjuvant therapy was found to remodel the pancreatic microenvironment by reversing the immunosuppressive behavior of cancer cells.[51] During carcinogenesis, pancreatic cancer cells promote regulatory T cells and myeloid-derived suppressor cells, which suppress the activity of effector cells. The immunosuppressive milieu is then promoted with dense desmoplastic reaction and sequestration of CD8+ T cells by activated pancreatic stellate cells. In this peritumoral niche, neoadjuvant therapy was shown to selectively deplete regulatory T cells and myeloid-derived suppressor cells, which ultimately correlated with enrichment of antitumor T cells, decreased stromal activation, and less neural invasion on histopathology.[51] Although PDAC is known to have low immunogenic potential, preconditioning of the tumor microenvironment with neoadjuvant chemotherapy may unleash a potentially effective immunotherapy response.

In summary, several studies have now demonstrated significant advantages of administrating neoadjuvant therapy, particularly in BR and LA pancreatic cancer, including higher margin negative resections, sterilization of regional lymph nodes, assessment of tumor biology and in vivo response, and more recently, as a guide to the receipt and type of adjuvant therapy. These benefits, however, have not been associated with a clear survival benefit over an adjuvant therapy approach on an intent to treat basis, particularly for resectable cancers. The assessment of biomarker response, however, either using traditional markers such as CA 19-9 or via liquid biopsies, coupled with an individualized approach to neoadjuvant therapy is anticipated to demonstrate survival benefits in the near future.

IRREVERSIBLE ELECTROPORATION

Approximately 30% of patients with PDAC present with LA (T4) unresectable disease due to encasement of the superior mesenteric artery, celiac axis, and/or a long segment of the hepatic artery, or occlusion of the superior mesenteric or portal vein without an option for vascular reconstruction.[7,52,53] Neoadjuvant chemoradiation may help with tumor regression, but only approximately 25% of the patients can be converted to resection, with 78% of those resected ultimately demonstrating negative margins in a meta-analysis of 325 patients with LA-PDAC.[38] For patients who remain unresectable after neoadjuvant therapy, locoregional therapy with IRE could provide a potential bridge to R0 resection and may increase survival by several months.[7,52]

To perform an IRE, needle electrodes (Fig. 2) are inserted into the PDAC and along the tumor periphery. These electrodes then emit high-voltage electrical pulses to disrupt plasma membrane permeability by creating nanopores thereby disrupting intracellular homeostasis and inducing cell apoptosis.[7] As IRE is a nonthermal local treatment, it is safe to use in this critical anatomic area. Although IRE can cause cancer cell death through apoptosis, it leaves protein structural matrices such as vascular elastin and collagen within the vessels and ducts intact so they can re-epithelize.[53,54] Thus, unlike other ablative techniques such as radiofrequency or microwave ablation, IRE can be applied to tumor edges adjacent to major vasculature, pancreatic duct, and bile duct without the morbidity of thermal injury.[7,53] This makes IRE a favorable modality for treating LA-PDACs that encase major vessels without being susceptible to vascular injury or heat sink effect.[53]

IRE can be performed via an open or laparoscopic surgery using ultrasound guidance for local tumor control and to extend surgical margins at the time of pancreatectomy, or it can be performed percutaneously using CT or ultrasound guidance.[53–55] For optimal results, IRE is recommended for PDAC tumors smaller than 3 to 5 cm.[52,53] When applied properly on pancreatic tissue, IRE generally uses 1400 to 2000 V/cm at a pulse length of 90 ms for a maximum of 270 pulses.[53] Inappropriate application of pulses, voltage, and interprobe distance may lead to complications.[53] In addition, presence of metals such as indwelling biliary stent, surgical clips, and fiducials within the ablation zone can cause deflection of energy and incomplete ablation.[53] After an IRE session, histologic changes of edema and hemorrhage may be evident as early as 30 min post-

Fig. 2. A pair of electrode probes are used to deliver a flow of current in the pancreatic tissue to disrupt plasma membrane. (*Image courtesy of* AngioDynamics, Inc. and its affiliates.)

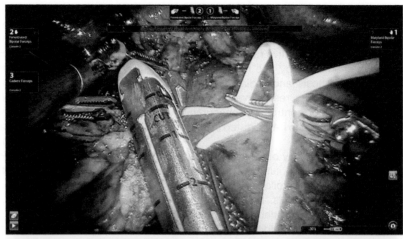

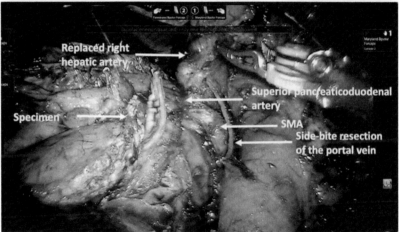

procedure as demonstrated in animal models, and with a clear ablation zone apparent in 7 to 14 days.[53] After 3 months, the tumor should no longer enhance on contrast imaging, as would be expected with a fibrotic scar.[53] Persistent enhancement should raise the concern for incomplete ablation or local recurrence.

In a systemic review of 18 original studies, outcomes of 498 patients with unresectable LA-PDAC were analyzed following IRE.[54] In total, 16% of patients achieved complete tumor remission and 38.2% achieved partial tumor response.[54] After IRE, 5.3% of patients were downstaged to undergo curative-intent operations.[54] Approximately 30% of patients had post-procedure complications, including 21% major complications, with a 2.2% mortality rate.[54] The median overall survival after IRE ranged from 7 to 27 months, and the median progression-free survival ranged from 5 to 15 months.[54] PDAC greater than 3 cm and those with early local progression within 6 months post-procedure were associated with worse prognosis.[54] The survival benefit following IRE remains to be elucidated as these studies had a heterogenous group of patients with variable regimens and amount of neoadjuvant therapy.

Recently, a multicenter, prospective, single-arm, phase II study (PANFIRE) was published to evaluate the efficacy and long-term safety of percutaneous IRE for 40 patients with LA-PDAC and 10 patients with isolated local recurrence after PDAC resection.[52] With IRE, the median overall survival was extended to 17 months for patients with LA-PDAC, and 16 months for patients with post-resection local recurrence.[52] Both of these median overall survivals exceeded the expected survival of patients receiving standard of care (9–14 months with gemcitabine-based or FOLFIRI-NOX therapy).[52] Complications occurred in 29 (58%) patients, including 21 (42%) patients who had major complications, with 2 (1%) deaths within 90 days after IRE.[52] These data need to be carefully weighed against the encouraging report by Memorial Sloan Kettering Cancer Cetner (MSKCC) on the use of hypofractionated ablative radiation therapy using 98 Gy biologically effective dose for LAPC.[56] In this cohort study of 119 consecutive patients with localized, unresectable PDAC treated with ablative radiation therapy after induction chemotherapy, the median overall survival from diagnosis and radiation therapy was 26.8 and 18.4 months, respectively.[56] This durable locoregional tumor control and encouraging survival outcomes need to be validated in prospective randomized trials.

In summary, IRE may offer survival benefits for patients with LA-PDAC, although future prospective randomized controlled trials are urgently needed to validate this benefit over modern chemotherapy and compare it to other locoregional treatments. In addition, IRE should be applied with caution given its not insignificant rates of morbidities and mortality.

SUMMARY

In conclusion, three major advancements in the surgical treatment of PDAC have emerged in the past decade that have significantly changed our modern-day surgical management of this aggressive disease. Each of these advances holds great promise in improving patient outcomes and survival but remain a matter of extensive investigation. Whether minimally invasive pancreatectomy can reduce operative morbidity, neoadjuvant therapy help improve survival, and IRE facilitate downstaging LA disease to resection will likely depend on careful patient selection and a multidisciplinary approach.

DISCLOSURE

The authors have nothing to disclose.

REFERENCES

1. Siegel RL, Miller KD, Fuchs HE, et al. Cancer Statistics, 2021. CA Cancer J Clin 2021;71(1):7–33.
2. Neoptolemos JP, Stocken DD, Dunn JA, et al. Influence of resection margins on survival for patients with pancreatic cancer treated by adjuvant chemoradiation and/or chemotherapy in the ESPAC-1 randomized controlled trial. Ann Surg 2001;234(6): 758–68.
3. Oettle H, Neuhaus P, Hochhaus A, et al. Adjuvant chemotherapy with gemcitabine and long-term outcomes among patients with resected pancreatic cancer: the CONKO-001 randomized trial. JAMA 2013;310(14):1473–81.
4. Neoptolemos JP, Palmer DH, Ghaneh P, et al. Comparison of adjuvant gemcitabine and capecitabine with gemcitabine monotherapy in patients with resected pancreatic cancer (ESPAC-4): a multicentre, open-label, randomised, phase 3 trial. Lancet 2017;389(10073):1011–24.
5. Conroy T, Hammel P, Hebbar M, et al. FOLFIRINOX or Gemcitabine as Adjuvant Therapy for Pancreatic Cancer. N Engl J Med 2018;379(25):2395–406.
6. van Hilst J, de Graaf N, Abu Hilal M, et al. The Landmark Series: Minimally Invasive Pancreatic Resection. Ann Surg Oncol 2021;28(3):1447–56.
7. van Rijssen LB, Rombouts SJ, Walma MS, et al. Recent Advances in Pancreatic Cancer Surgery of Relevance to the Practicing Pathologist. Surg Pathol Clin 2016;9(4):539–45.
8. Kneuertz PJ, Patel SH, Chu CK, et al. Effects of perioperative red blood cell transfusion on disease recurrence and survival after pancreaticoduodenectomy for ductal adenocarcinoma. Ann Surg Oncol 2011;18(5):1327–34.
9. Girgis MD, Zenati MS, King JC, et al. Oncologic Outcomes After Robotic Pancreatic Resections Are Not Inferior to Open Surgery. Ann Surg 2019. https://doi.org/10.1097/SLA.0000000000003615.
10. Beane JD, Zenati M, Hamad A, et al. Robotic pancreatoduodenectomy with vascular resection: Outcomes and learning curve. Surgery 2019;166(1):8–14.
11. Croome KP, Farnell MB, Que FG, et al. Pancreaticoduodenectomy with major vascular resection: a comparison of laparoscopic versus open approaches. J Gastrointest Surg 2015;19(1):189–94, [discussion: 194].
12. Beane JD, Pitt HA, Dolejs SC, et al. Assessing the impact of conversion on outcomes of minimally invasive distal pancreatectomy and pancreatoduodenectomy. HPB (Oxford) 2018;20(4):356–63.
13. Zureikat AH, Borrebach J, Pitt HA, et al. Minimally invasive hepatopancreatobiliary surgery in North America: an ACS-NSQIP analysis of predictors of conversion for laparoscopic and robotic pancreatectomy and hepatectomy. HPB (Oxford) 2017; 19(7):595–602.
14. Nassour I, Wang SC, Christie A, et al. Minimally Invasive Versus Open Pancreaticoduodenectomy: A Propensity-matched Study From a National Cohort of Patients. Ann Surg 2018;268(1):151–7.
15. Palanivelu C, Senthilnathan P, Sabnis SC, et al. Randomized clinical trial of laparoscopic versus open pancreatoduodenectomy for periampullary tumours. Br J Surg 2017;104(11):1443–50.
16. Poves I, Burdio F, Morato O, et al. Comparison of Perioperative Outcomes Between Laparoscopic and Open Approach for Pancreatoduodenectomy: The PADULAP Randomized Controlled Trial. Ann Surg 2018;268(5):731–9.
17. de Rooij T, van Hilst J, Bosscha K, et al. Minimally invasive versus open pancreatoduodenectomy (LEOPARD-2): study protocol for a randomized controlled trial. Trials 2018;19(1):1.

18. van Hilst J, de Rooij T, Bosscha K, et al. Laparoscopic versus open pancreatoduodenectomy for pancreatic or periampullary tumours (LEOPARD-2): a multicentre, patient-blinded, randomised controlled phase 2/3 trial. Lancet Gastroenterol Hepatol 2019;4(3):199–207.

19. Wang M, Li D, Chen R, et al. Laparoscopic versus open pancreatoduodenectomy for pancreatic or periampullary tumours: a multicentre, open-label, randomised controlled trial. Lancet Gastroenterol Hepatol 2021;6(6):438–47.

20. Boone BA, Zenati M, Hogg ME, et al. Assessment of quality outcomes for robotic pancreaticoduodenectomy: identification of the learning curve. JAMA Surg 2015;150(5):416–22.

21. Asbun HJ, Moekotte AL, Vissers FL, et al. The Miami International Evidence-based Guidelines on Minimally Invasive Pancreas Resection. Ann Surg 2020;271(1):1–14.

22. Zureikat AH, Postlewait LM, Liu Y, et al. A Multi-institutional Comparison of Perioperative Outcomes of Robotic and Open Pancreaticoduodenectomy. Ann Surg 2016;264(4):640–9.

23. Nassour I, Winters SB, Hoehn R, et al. Long-term oncologic outcomes of robotic and open pancreatectomy in a national cohort of pancreatic adenocarcinoma. J Surg Oncol 2020;122(2):234–42.

24. de Rooij T, van Hilst J, van Santvoort H, et al. Minimally Invasive Versus Open Distal Pancreatectomy (LEOPARD): A Multicenter Patient-blinded Randomized Controlled Trial. Ann Surg 2019;269(1):2–9.

25. Bjornsson B, Larsson AL, Hjalmarsson C, et al. Comparison of the duration of hospital stay after laparoscopic or open distal pancreatectomy: randomized controlled trial. Br J Surg 2020;107(10):1281–8.

26. Neoptolemos JP, Dunn JA, Stocken DD, et al. Adjuvant chemoradiotherapy and chemotherapy in resectable pancreatic cancer: a randomised controlled trial. Lancet 2001;358(9293):1576–85.

27. Neoptolemos JP, Moore MJ, Cox TF, et al. Effect of adjuvant chemotherapy with fluorouracil plus folinic acid or gemcitabine vs observation on survival in patients with resected periampullary adenocarcinoma: the ESPAC-3 periampullary cancer randomized trial. JAMA 2012;308(2):147–56.

28. Ahmad SA, Duong M, Sohal DPS, et al. Surgical Outcome Results From SWOG S1505: A Randomized Clinical Trial of mFOLFIRINOX Versus Gemcitabine/Nab-paclitaxel for Perioperative Treatment of Resectable Pancreatic Ductal Adenocarcinoma. Ann Surg 2020;272(3):481–6.

29. Patel SH, Katz MHG, Ahmad SA. The Landmark Series: Preoperative Therapy for Pancreatic Cancer. Ann Surg Oncol 2021;28(8):4104–29.

30. Raufi AG, Manji GA, Chabot JA, et al. Neoadjuvant Treatment for Pancreatic Cancer. Semin Oncol 2019;46(1):19–27.

31. Versteijne E, Suker M, Groothuis K, et al. Preoperative Chemoradiotherapy Versus Immediate Surgery for Resectable and Borderline Resectable Pancreatic Cancer: Results of the Dutch Randomized Phase III PREOPANC Trial. J Clin Oncol 2020; 38(16):1763–73.

32. Evans DB, Varadhachary GR, Crane CH, et al. Preoperative gemcitabine-based chemoradiation for patients with resectable adenocarcinoma of the pancreatic head. J Clin Oncol 2008;26(21): 3496–502.

33. Pisters PW, Abbruzzese JL, Janjan NA, et al. Rapid-fractionation preoperative chemoradiation, pancreaticoduodenectomy, and intraoperative radiation therapy for resectable pancreatic adenocarcinoma. J Clin Oncol 1998;16(12):3843–50.

34. Pisters PW, Wolff RA, Janjan NA, et al. Preoperative paclitaxel and concurrent rapid-fractionation radiation for resectable pancreatic adenocarcinoma: toxicities, histologic response rates, and event-free outcome. J Clin Oncol 2002;20(10): 2537–44.

35. Jang JY, Han Y, Lee H, et al. Oncological Benefits of Neoadjuvant Chemoradiation With Gemcitabine Versus Upfront Surgery in Patients With Borderline Resectable Pancreatic Cancer: A Prospective, Randomized, Open-label, Multicenter Phase 2/3 Trial. Ann Surg 2018;268(2):215–22.

36. Murphy JE, Wo JY, Ryan DP, et al. Total Neoadjuvant Therapy With FOLFIRINOX Followed by Individualized Chemoradiotherapy for Borderline Resectable Pancreatic Adenocarcinoma: A Phase 2 Clinical Trial. JAMA Oncol 2018;4(7):963–9.

37. Marthey L, Sa-Cunha A, Blanc JF, et al. FOLFIRINOX for locally advanced pancreatic adenocarcinoma: results of an AGEO multicenter prospective observational cohort. Ann Surg Oncol 2015;22(1): 295–301.

38. Suker M, Beumer BR, Sadot E, et al. FOLFIRINOX for locally advanced pancreatic cancer: a systematic review and patient-level meta-analysis. Lancet Oncol 2016;17(6):801–10.

39. Sohal DPS, Duong M, Ahmad SA, et al. Efficacy of Perioperative Chemotherapy for Resectable Pancreatic Adenocarcinoma: A Phase 2 Randomized Clinical Trial. JAMA Oncol 2021;7(3):421–7.

40. Tempero MA, Malafa MP, Chiorean EG, et al. Pancreatic Adenocarcinoma, Version 1.2019. J Natl Compr Canc Netw 2019;17(3):202–10.

41. Tzeng CW, Tran Cao HS, Lee JE, et al. Treatment sequencing for resectable pancreatic cancer: influence of early metastases and surgical complications on multimodality therapy completion and survival. J Gastrointest Surg 2014;18(1):16–24, [discussion: 24–5].

42. Merkow RP, Bilimoria KY, Tomlinson JS, et al. Postoperative complications reduce adjuvant

chemotherapy use in resectable pancreatic cancer. Ann Surg 2014;260(2):372–7.

43. Adam MA, Nassour I, Hoehn R, et al. Neoadjuvant Chemotherapy for Pancreatic Adenocarcinoma Lessens the Deleterious Effect of Omission of Adjuvant Chemotherapy. Ann Surg Oncol 2021;28(7): 3800–7.

44. Tsai S, George B, Wittmann D, et al. Importance of Normalization of CA19-9 Levels Following Neoadjuvant Therapy in Patients With Localized Pancreatic Cancer. Ann Surg 2020;271(4):740–7.

45. Macedo FI, Ryon E, Maithel SK, et al. Survival Outcomes Associated With Clinical and Pathological Response Following Neoadjuvant FOLFIRINOX or Gemcitabine/Nab-Paclitaxel Chemotherapy in Resected Pancreatic Cancer. Ann Surg 2019;270(3): 400–13.

46. Liu H, Zenati MS, Rieser CJ, et al. CA19-9 Change During Neoadjuvant Therapy May Guide the Need for Additional Adjuvant Therapy Following Resected Pancreatic Cancer. Ann Surg Oncol 2020;27(10): 3950–60.

47. Martens S, Lefesvre P, Nicolle R, et al. Different shades of pancreatic ductal adenocarcinoma, different paths towards precision therapeutic applications. Ann Oncol 2019;30(9):1428–36.

48. Moffitt RA, Marayati R, Flate EL, et al. Virtual microdissection identifies distinct tumor- and stroma-specific subtypes of pancreatic ductal adenocarcinoma. Nat Genet 2015;47(10):1168–78.

49. Imamura M, Nagayama M, Kyuno D, et al. Perioperative Predictors of Early Recurrence for Resectable and Borderline-Resectable Pancreatic Cancer. Cancers 2021;13(10). https://doi.org/10.3390/cancers13102285.

50. Gemenetzis G, Groot VP, Yu J, et al. Circulating Tumor Cells Dynamics in Pancreatic Adenocarcinoma Correlate With Disease Status: Results of the Prospective CLUSTER Study. Ann Surg 2018;268(3): 408–20.

51. Mota Reyes C, Teller S, Muckenhuber A, et al. Neoadjuvant Therapy Remodels the Pancreatic Cancer Microenvironment via Depletion of Protumorigenic Immune Cells. Clin Cancer Res 2020;26(1):220–31.

52. Ruarus AH, Vroomen L, Geboers B, et al. Percutaneous Irreversible Electroporation in Locally Advanced and Recurrent Pancreatic Cancer (PANFIRE-2): A Multicenter, Prospective, Single-Arm, Phase II Study. Radiology 2020;294(1):212–20.

53. Rashid MF, Hecht EM, Steinman JA, et al. Irreversible electroporation of pancreatic adenocarcinoma: a primer for the radiologist. Abdom Radiol (NY) 2018;43(2):457–66.

54. Moris D, Machairas N, Tsilimigras DI, et al. Systematic Review of Surgical and Percutaneous Irreversible Electroporation in the Treatment of Locally Advanced Pancreatic Cancer. Ann Surg Oncol 2019;26(6):1657–68.

55. Kwon W, Thomas A, Kluger MD. Irreversible electroporation of locally advanced pancreatic cancer. Semin Oncol 2021. https://doi.org/10.1053/j.seminoncol.2021.02.004.

56. Reyngold M, O'Reilly EM, Varghese AM, et al. Association of Ablative Radiation Therapy With Survival Among Patients With Inoperable Pancreatic Cancer. JAMA Oncol 2021;7(5):735–8.

The Evolving Paradigm of Germline Testing in Pancreatic Ductal Adenocarcinoma and Implications for Clinical Practice

Chirayu Mohindroo, MD[a,b], Ana De Jesus-Acosta, MD[c],
Matthew B. Yurgelun, MD[d], Anirban Maitra, MD[e],
Maureen Mork, MS, CGC[f], Florencia McAllister, MD[a,f,g,h],*

KEYWORDS

- Pancreatic ductal adenocarcinoma • Germline mutations • Cancer screening
- Multigene panel testing • Genetic testing • PARP inhibitors • Immunotherapy

Key points

- Recent studies have shown prevalence of pathogenic germline mutations in pancreatic ductal adenocarcinoma (PDAC) patients not selected for any traditional high-risk features can be as high as 8% to 10%.
- Both National Comprehensive Cancer Network and American Society of Clinical Oncology now recommend universal germline testing in PDAC patients.
- Presence of germline mutations can have a significant clinical impact owing to targeted therapies, which are now considered standard of care in such individuals.
- Genetic testing in PDAC patients has also helped to identify mutation-positive relatives, a high-risk group that would benefit from PDAC screening.

ABSTRACT

Identification of deleterious germline mutations in pancreatic ductal adenocarcinoma (PDAC) patients can have therapeutic implications for the patients and result in cascade testing and prevention in their relatives. Universal testing for germline mutations is now considered standard of care in patients with PDAC, regardless of family history, personal history, or age. Here, we highlight the commonly identified germline mutations in PDAC patients as well as the impact of multigene panel testing. We further discuss therapeutic implications of germline testing on the index cases, and the impact of cascade testing on cancer early detection and prevention in relatives.

[a] Department of Clinical Cancer Prevention, The University of Texas MD Anderson Cancer Center, 1515 Holcombe, Unit 1360, Houston, TX 77030, USA; [b] Department of Internal Medicine, Sinai Hospital of Baltimore, 2435 W. Belvedere Ave, Ste 56, Baltimore, MD 21215, USA; [c] Department of Oncology, The Sidney Kimmel Comprehensive Cancer Center at Johns Hopkins, Johns Hopkins University School of Medicine, 401 North Broadway, Baltimore, MD 21231, USA; [d] Department of Medical Oncology, Dana-Farber Cancer Institute, 450 Brookline Avenue, Boston, MA 02215, USA; [e] Department of Translational Molecular Pathology, Sheikh Ahmed Center for Pancreatic Cancer Research, The University of Texas MD Anderson Cancer Center, 2130 West Holcombe Boulevard, Houston, TX 77030, USA; [f] Clinical Cancer Genetics Program, The University of Texas MD Anderson Cancer Center, 1515 Holcombe, Houston, TX 77030, USA; [g] Department of Gastrointestinal Medical Oncology, The University of Texas MD Anderson Cancer Center, Houston, TX, USA; [h] Department of Immunology, The University of Texas MD Anderson Cancer Center, Houston, TX, USA
* Corresponding author. Department of Clinical Cancer Prevention, The University of Texas MD Anderson Cancer Center, 1515 Holcombe, Unit 1360, Houston, TX, 77030, United States
E-mail address: FMcallister@mdanderson.org

Surgical Pathology 15 (2022) 491–502
https://doi.org/10.1016/j.path.2022.05.004

surgpath.theclinics.com

OVERVIEW

In 2022, it is estimated that there will be 62,210 new cases of pancreatic cancer, and approximately 49,380 people will die of this disease. Pancreatic ductal adenocarcinoma, or PDAC, is the most common subtype of pancreatic cancer, accounting for greater than 95% of pancreatic neoplasms, and the 2 terms will be used interchangeably for the purposes of this commentary. The 5-year survival rate of PDAC is 11%, making it the third most common cause of cancer-related death in the United States.[1] The dismal prognosis of the disease can be attributed to the inability of early detection and the absence of effective therapy. Identification of germline mutations can provide critical insights on targeted therapies or immunotherapy. The most common susceptibility genes associated with higher risk for pancreatic cancer include BReast CAncer gene 1 (BRCA1), BReast CAncer gene 2 (BRCA2), Ataxia Telangiectasia Mutated (ATM), Adenomatous Polyposis Coli (APC), Tumor Protein p53 (TP53), Partner And Localizer Of BRCA2 (PALB2), Cyclin Dependent Kinase Inhibitor 2A (CDKN2A), Serine/Threonine Kinase 11 (STK11), MutL Homolog 1 (MLH1), MutS Homolog 2 (MSH2), MutS Homolog 6 (MSH6), and EPithelial Cellular Adhesion Molecule (EPCAM).[2] These genes confer variable degree of increased risk for PDAC and also confer susceptibility to other cancer types.

Studies have reported a prevalence of germline mutations ranging from 4% to 20% in PDAC patients.[3–9] This considerable variation is likely due to differences not only in the specific panel of genes tested in each study but also in geographic variations, racial composition, and other demographic features such as age of the tested cohorts or Ashkenazi Jewish background. Advances in next-generation sequencing have expanded the panel of genes that are interrogated within available multigene assays. Therefore, the highest reported prevalence of 20% comes from Goldstein and colleagues and Lowery and colleagues,[7,10] testing for 263 genes and 76 genes, respectively, in unselected cohorts; however, not all mutations identified were in genes well-associated with PDAC risk. Recent studies have revealed that PDAC patients lacking distinct high-risk features such as strong family history can be carriers of germline mutations and patients with family history of PDAC do not have higher prevalence of mutations.[11,12] This accumulating evidence led to the change in National Comprehensive Cancer Network (NCCN) guidelines, which now recommend germline testing for all PDAC patients.[13]

Treatment decisions based on germline testing results can improve clinical outcomes. A recent publication stated that PDAC patients with a somatic or germline mutation who received therapy matched to their mutations exhibited an increase of 1 year median overall survival (OS) as compared with those patients who received standard-of-care therapy.[14] Poly-ADP (adenosine diphosphate)-ribose polymerase (PARP) inhibitors can target BRCA1, BRCA2, PALB2, and potentially ATM carriers. A hallmark study by Golan and colleagues reported that metastatic PDAC patients with germline BRCA1/BRCA2 mutations had almost doubling of the progression-free survival with maintenance therapy using PARP inhibitor olaparib.[15] This led to the FDA approval of olaparib,[16] and various clinical trials are now evaluating the efficacy of other PARP inhibitors as monotherapy or in combination with other agents in patients with DNA damage repair (DDR) gene defects.[17,18] Immunotherapy, which has been incredibly responsive in patients harboring mismatch repair (MMR)-related germline mutations in other cancers,[19] has failed to demonstrate efficacy in PDAC patients.[20,21] However, combination with another immunotherapy agent[22] and other modalities such as chemotherapy[23,24] and radiotherapy has been promising.[25] Besides targeted therapy, Bannon and colleagues showed PDAC patients with germline mutations, regardless of the treatment received, were found to have better survival outcomes, indicating that germline mutations could also serve as a prognostic marker.[11]

Germline testing has also proven helpful for cascade testing in close relatives of PDAC patients. This can lead to identifying currently asymptomatic relatives with germline mutations conferring higher risk for PDAC who would be eligible for surveillance.[26,27] Several high-risk screening programs have been developed across institutions, and data about benefit of screening are now being reported.[1,28] Screening this high-risk population using endoscopic ultrasound/MRI has led to detection of PDAC (or even high-grade precursor lesions) at early stages.[29–31] Besides screening for PDAC, healthy individuals found to harbor germline mutations can also be recommended syndrome-specific interventions for prevention or early detection of other cancers.

This article reviews prominent studies that have established the frequency and type of germline mutations reported in PDAC patients, includes descriptions of the most common mutations, highlights the importance of multigene panel testing, and describes its impact on targeted therapies and screening.

GERMLINE MUTATION IN PANCREATIC DUCTAL ADENOCARCINOMA

DNA DAMAGE REPAIR GENES (BRCA1/BRCA2/PALB2/ATM)

BRCA1 and *BRCA2* genes encode for tumor suppressor proteins that are involved in repairing double-strand DNA breaks via the homologous DNA repair mechanism. Pathogenetic germline mutations within *BRCA1* and *BRCA2* are known to increase risk for breast and ovarian cancer. These deleterious mutations are now known to be a risk factor for the development of PDAC and were identified as deleterious in PDAC patients in the 1990s. This early association was made when a study reported that 3 out of 41 patients had a *BRCA2* germline mutation in an unselected cohort of PDAC patients.[32] Presence of germline mutations in *BRCA1/BRCA2* in patients with PDAC is estimated to be about 5% to 9%.[7,33,34] The frequency is higher in certain groups such as familial pancreatic cancer as high as 17%[35–37] and in Ashkenazi Jews up to 21%.[6,12,17,28,38] Even with multigene panel testing *BRCA1/BRCA2* seem to be the most frequently identified germline mutations in PDAC patients. *BRCA2* being much more common ranging from 5.2%[7] to 1.34%,[3] whereas the prevalence for *BRCA1* ranges from 2.4%[7] to 0.35%.[12]

PALB2 (Partner and Localizer of BRCA2) is a DNA repair gene that has been associated with increased risk of PDAC. Jones and colleagues via exomic sequencing first identified *PALB2* as a pancreatic cancer susceptibility gene.[39] The *PALB2* gene produces a protein that functions as a tumor suppressor by interacting with both BRCA1 and BRCA2 during double-strand DNA repair.[40] Boreck and colleagues reported that *PALB2* germline mutations represented 2% of an unselected PDAC patient cohort.[41] Most of the multigene panel studies subsequently reported a prevalence between 0.76%[8] and 0.23%.[12]

ATM serine/threonine kinase (*ATM*) is part of the phosphoinositide 3-kinase-related protein kinase family.[42] *ATM* plays a role in the signaling required to initiate DNA repair, and thus, *ATM* defects can lead to genomic instability and higher risk of cancer development.[42–44] Iconic study comes from Roberts and colleagues, who performed sequence analysis of 166 familial PDAC probands, identifying 2.4% individuals carrying pathogenic *ATM* mutations.[43] *ATM* has been consistently found in various multigene panels in PDAC, with a prevalence ranging from 1.02%[8] to as high as 3.35%[3] in unselected cohorts.

A study worth highlighting in would be by Yurgelun and colleagues, which showed a prognostic benefit in patients who tested positive for mutations in DDR genes. The unselected cohort consisting of 289 patients found a statistically significant and superior OS in carriers of DNA damage response gene mutations when compared with noncarriers, with median OS of 34.4 versus 19.1 months, in the 28 (9.7%) patients with double-strand DNA damage repair mutations compared with noncarriers.[9]

DNA MISMATCH REPAIR GENES (MLH1/MLH2/MSH6)

Microsatellites are repeat sequences that are scattered throughout the genome between coding and noncoding sequences. These alterations are corrected postreplication by the DNA MMR process. Defects in MMR lead to genomic instability, particularly affecting repeat regions and giving rise to the microsatellite instability-high (MSI-H) phenotype.[45] MSI can occur in tumors either at a somatic level or via germline mutations in one of the MMR genes (*MLH1*, *MSH2*, *MSH6*). Lynch syndrome is associated with an increased risk of colorectal and other gastrointestinal tract-related neoplasms, including pancreatic cancer, as well as endometrial and other cancers. Lynch syndrome patients have almost a 9-fold higher risk of PDAC in comparison to the general population and varies depending on the causative gene.[46,47] The prevalence for mutations in these genes has generally been found to be less than 1%, ranging from 0.03%[6] to 0.69%[9] across the multigene tested PDAC cohorts. Similar to other cancers, having MSI in PDAC can have substantial diagnostic and therapeutic implications.[48,49]

CDKN2A

CDKN2A is a tumor suppressor gene classically associated with familial atypical multiple mole and melanoma syndrome. Pathogenic alterations in the *CDKN2A* gene have also been associated with increased risk of PDAC. An earlier study focused on this mutation reported 9 (0.6%) cases in an unselected cohort of 1537 cases.[50] More recent multigene studies have found *CDKN2A* mutations in unselected cohorts as well, with a prevalence ranging from 0.11%[12] to 0.97%.[7] Furthermore, in a retrospective evaluation of 568 individuals at high risk for PDAC, *CDKN2A-p16-Leiden* mutation carriers was the only group found to harbor a substantial number of PDAC cases.[51]

TP53

TP53 is a tumor suppressor gene associated with cell cycle regulation. Li-Fraumeni syndrome is the hereditary condition associated with mutations in *TP53*. The gene has also been associated with increased risk of PDAC and was part of the multi-gene panels of most major studies conducted. The prevalence has been found to be as high as 0.75% in PDAC unselected cohorts.[10]

STK11/LKB1

Mutations in the *STK11/LKB1* tumor suppressor gene located on chromosome 19p13.3 lead to an autosomal dominant disorder known as Peutz-Jeghers syndrome (PJS).[52–54] The syndrome is associated with gastrointestinal tract polyposis along with an increased risk for breast, gastrointestinal tract, and gynecologic cancers, with the specific risk of PDAC determined to be 132-fold higher than the general population.[55] Furthermore, in a multicenter study conducted in patients with PJS, the risk of developing PDAC was determined to be the highest of any other gene.[56] Our group has reported a successful case of early detection and cancer interception in a patient with PJS who was found to have a premalignant lesion while undergoing screening.[57]

GENES ASSOCIATED WITH CHRONIC/HEREDITARY PANCREATITIS

Chronic pancreatitis has been associated with mutations *PRSS1*, *SPINK1*, *CTRC*, and *CFTR*.[58] Long-standing chronic inflammation does increase the risk of developing PDAC, ranging from 7%[59] to 20%.[60] The most robust evidence comes from a 20-year prospective study, where the risk associated with PDAC was calculated to be 7.2%.[59] However, the results have not been consistent.[61,62] In a meta-analysis consisting of 11 case control studies, results showed a modest increase with the *CFTR* gene and no association was found with *SPINK1*.[58] These genes are usually not screened in the absence of personal or family history of chronic pancreatitis.

IMPACT OF MULTIGENE PANEL TESTING

In recent years, there has been a dramatic increase in the use of multigene panel testing in PDAC. Multigene panel testing via next-generation sequencing (NGS) technologies has allowed us to simultaneously test for multiple genes. Targeted single-gene analysis may still be suitable when testing an individual from a family with a known pathogenic variant.[63] In cases when more than one gene may explain a patient's clinical presentation and family history, selecting a multigene panel testing may be more beneficial, as compared with targeted single-gene testing.[64] Multigene panel testing allows not only for the identification of pathogenic alterations in genes associated with the patient phenotype but also for the identification of incidental pathogenic variants not suspected based on patient personal or family history.[65]

These features make multigene panel testing particularly relevant in the context of PDAC. A study conducted by Mandelker and colleagues reported that a genetic testing strategy focused only on family history, personal history, age, and ethnicity would miss approximately 42% of individuals with a pathogenic germline alteration in PDAC,[66] along with various unselected PDAC cohorts reporting high germline mutation prevalence in PDAC patients, led to the NCCN guidelines recommending universal germline testing in all individuals diagnosed with PDAC.[13]

There is no specific recommendation as to which genes need to be included in the panel, although the NCCN does mention *BRCA1*, *BRCA2*, *PALB2*, *ATM*, *CDKN2A*, *MSH2*, *MSH6*, *MLH1*, *EPCAM*, *TP53*, and *STK11* as the ones that should be included.[67] New studies do favor increasing the number of genes to be included on multigene panels. As shown in **Fig. 1**A, germline mutation prevalence does increase with higher number of genes tested. It is also important to note that the difference in techniques could increase the prevalence, as Goldstein and colleagues used targeted exome sequencing, which revealed novel germline mutations; therefore, they reported a prevalence higher prevalence in a smaller cohort (N = 133) as compared with other studies.[10] As mentioned earlier, although checking a larger number of genes does seem to increase the prevalence of germline mutations in PDAC, it does not necessarily establish causality.

The commonly tested genes along with the percentages are reported in **Fig. 1**B, **Supplementary Table 1**, **Supplementary Table 2**.

Despite the impact of multigene panel testing for individuals with PDAC, it is also important to acknowledge its limitations. Multigene panels can identify pathogenic variants for which clinical management is unclear due to the lack of data pertaining to cancer risk along with the increased risk of finding variants of uncertain significance that are not actionable.[63,68] This has also further complicated genetic counseling; if skilled genetic counseling is not given, besides anxiety for the patient and family members, it may lead to over-treatment or overscreening.[69] Limiting the number of genes evaluated under the guidance of appropriate expertise may help tackle these challenges.[68,69]

Fig. 1. (*A*) Prevalence of germline mutations across unselected study Groups. (*B*) Graphical representation of individual genes prevalence across unselected cohorts.

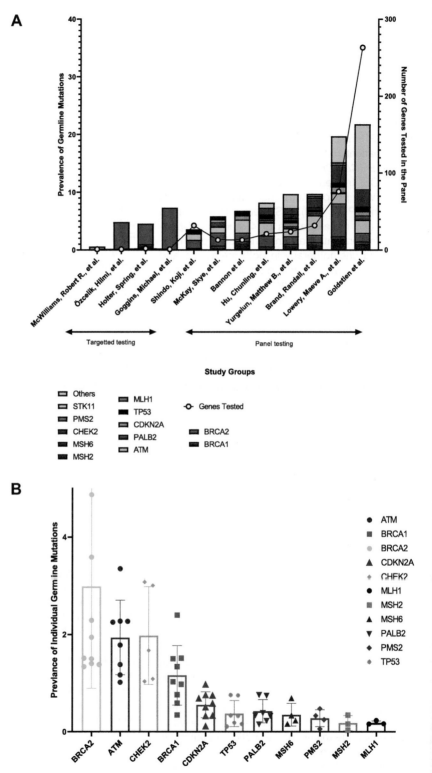

TARGETED THERAPY IN PATIENTS WITH GERMLINE MUTATIONS

The treatment response for patients with PDAC with germline mutations has been well studied with DNA repair genes (BRCA1, BRCA2, and PALB2) in the context of platinum-containing chemotherapy agents and benefit from treatment with PARP inhibitors. In a retrospective study, 71 PDAC patients (stages III/IV) with germline mutations in BRCA1/BRCA2 were found to have a superior OS treated with platinum versus those treated with nonplatinum chemotherapies (22 vs 9 months; $P = .039$).[70] Systemic review of 16 studies and meta-analysis of 4 studies, respectively, demonstrated a benefit in using platinum-containing chemotherapy in both metastatic and resected cohorts of PDAC patients with homologous recombination deficiency (both germline and somatic).[71] NCCN now recommends platinum-based chemotherapy such as FOLinic acid , Fluorouracil, IRINotecan hydrochloride, and OXaliplatin (FOLFIRINOX) or cisplatin combined with gemcitabine hydrochloride as first-line treatment of patients with PDAC, who have good performance status, and known germline mutations in BRCA1/BRCA2 or PALB2.[13]

Recently, PARP Inhibitors have also shown promising therapeutic benefit in patients with PDAC and germline mutations in DNA repair genes.[72] Convincing evidence of PARP inhibition comes from the phase III POLO trial in advanced PDAC patients.[15] The study population consisted of patients with germline BRCA1/BRCA2-mutated advanced PDAC who had not progressed on platinum-based first-line chemotherapy ($\geq$16 weeks) and received either olaparib as maintenance treatment or placebo. In the intervention arm, olaparib nearly doubled the median PFS compared with placebo (7.4 vs 3.8 months; $P = .004$), whereas OS remained similar in both arms (18.9 vs 18.1 months; $P = .68$).[15] This led to the FDA approval of olaparib in patients with deleterious or suspected deleterious germline BRCA1/BRCA2-mutated metastatic PDAC.[16] Another single-arm phase II trial using rucaparib as maintenance therapy after platinum-based induction demonstrated an objective response rate (ORR) of 37% with minimal toxicities in 19 advanced PDAC patients with a pathogenic germline or somatic mutation in BRCA1, BRCA2, or PALB2.[17] However, a phase II trial with gemcitabine/cisplatin and veliparib in patients with PDAC and germline mutations in BRCA1/BRCA2/PALB2 failed to demonstrate any additional benefit with veliparib (OS 15.5 months vs 16.4 months, $P = .6$).[73]

Rucaparib,[18] olaparib,[74] and veliparib[17] have been studied as second-line monotherapy in the same population but the results have been conflicting. Although veliparib monotherapy showed no objective responses,[17] other studies with olaparib and rucaparib have shown modest clinical benefit. Olaparib has an ORR of 22% (5 out of 23)[74] and rucaparib showed a disease control rate of 32% (6 out of 19).[73] Preclinical evidence also exists for RAD51C-deficient cells, which were found to be sensitive to olaparib.[75] APOLLO trial (NCT04858334) a randomized, double-blind study is now evaluating olaparib following adjuvant platinum-based chemotherapy in resected PDAC patients carrying pathogenic BRCA1, BRCA2, or PALB2 mutations.[76]

Targeted therapy for the ATM gene has not been established but the role has been evaluated with radiation therapy, chemotherapy, and agents exploiting targeting DNA repair.[77] Javle and colleagues conducted 2 parallel nonrandomized phase 2 clinical trials using olaparib in advanced PDAC patients, which had 7 patients with germline ATM mutations, showing significantly prolonged PFS compared with patients enrolled solely based on family history.[78] Ayers and colleagues showed 3 pancreatic cancer cell lines using ATM-targeting Short Hairpin RNA (shRNA) had significant sensitivity to radiation therapy but not to the chemotherapeutics tested, namely gemcitabine, topotecan, doxorubicin, olaparib, trametenib, cisplatin, mitomycin c, an ATR inhibitor (Ve821), and a DNA-Pkcs inhibitor (Nu7441).[79] Preclinical evidence also suggests that ATM inhibition via innate immune response in PDAC, which is further enhanced by radiation increases sensitivity to anti–PD-L1 therapy.[80] Other potential targets in patients with PDAC include proteins downstream of ATM, such as ATR and CHK1/2.[77] Clinical trials exploring the combination of gemcitabine with ATR inhibitors (NCT04616534),[81] CHK1 inhibitors (NCT02632448),[82] and WEE1 inhibitors (NCT02037230)[83] are now being conducted.

Similar to other cancers, germline mutations in DNA MMR genes and associated MSI in individuals with PDAC could potentially have a high response rates to immune checkpoint inhibitors. From 5 single-arm multicohort multicenter KEYNOTE trials number 012, 16, 028, 158, and 164, FDA approved pembrolizumab immunotherapy for solid tumors with MMR deficiency or MSI-H.[49,84] However, results with monotherapy with immune check point inhibitors have been suboptimal in PDAC patients,[20] likely related to the unique immunosuppressive tumor microenvironment. A phase II trial evaluated the efficacy of monotherapy regardless of the MSI status with Ipi-limumab in 27 patients with advanced PDAC, failed to demonstrate any clinical benefit.[21] The KEYNOTE-158 trial, specifically reported the effi-cacy of pembrolizumab in dMMR/MSI-H PDAC (n = 22) showing a clinical benefit.[85] It would be interesting to see the results of clinical trials (NCT02628067, NCT03849469, NCT04007744, NCT03871959) evaluating immunotherapy based on MSI status in PDAC patients.[86–89]

Combination with another immunotherapeutic agent or other modalities such as chemotherapy or radiation has also shown encouraging results. A phase 2 randomized clinical trial, consisting of 65 metastatic PDAC patients undergoing durvalu-mab plus tremelimumab therapy, showed a better ORR compared with durvalumab monotherapy.[22] Combination of immunotherapy with chemothera-peutic agents such as gemcitabine[23,90,91] or nab-paclitaxel[24] has shown more promising results.

IMPACT OF GERMLINE MUTATIONS ON SCREENING FOR PANCREATIC DUCTAL ADENOCARCINOMA

The US Preventive Services Task Force does not recommend routine screening for PDAC; however, surveillance is recommended for high-risk popula-tions.[92] Based on the latest NCCN guidelines, PDAC screening in high-risk individuals should be performed at experienced high-volume centers af-ter shared decision-making with the individuals about potential limitations of screening such as cost and the high incidence of benign or indetermi-nate pancreatic abnormalities. The recommenda-tions for screening differ based on age and family history. Briefly, individuals harboring mutations in ATM, BRCA1, BRCA2, MLH1, MSH2, MSH6, EPCAM, PALB2, and TP53 are recommended screening only with a positive family history of PDAC, whereas screening is recommended at an earlier age and regardless of family history in pa-tients with STK11 or CDKN2A mutations.[93] The ev-idence comes from numerous studies conducted in by multidisciplinary teams in a research setting showing the potential benefits of surveillance.

In a prospective study by Overbeek and col-leagues, among 366 individuals at high risk for PDAC, 10 individuals developed PDAC, all of whom had germline mutations: 7 in CDKN2A, 2 in STK11, and 1 in BRCA2.[94] In another study done across 3 centers of Europe, among 411 high-risk individuals, 15 developed PDAC, including 13 individuals with CDKN2A mutations and 1 with a BRCA2 mutation.[29] Canto and col-leagues screened a high-risk cohort of 354

individuals, out of which 14 developed PDAC and 1 of them was a BRCA1/BRCA2/PALB2 germline mutation carrier.[31]

Recently, the Genetic Education, Risk Assess-ment, and Testing study aimed to identify patho-genic variants in first-degree or second-degree relatives of PDAC patients with and without germ-line mutations, thereby providing the opportunity for early detection and interception of PDAC and other associated cancers. The study randomized the subjects to 2 remote methods of genetic edu-cation to determine how effective each method is at increasing enrollment in genetic testing.[95] Pre-liminary data has been promising with both the arms of enrollment, showing genetic testing up-take rates up to 92% and a high rate of identifica-tion of germline pathogenic variant carriers, who may benefit from PDAC screening.[27]

SUMMARY

Germline testing has had a significant impact on the management of PDAC, in terms of treatment, diagnosis, and screening. Testing for germline mu-tations in BRCA1/BRCA2 and PALB2 is recom-mended to identify patients who may potentially benefit from platinum-based chemotherapy regi-mens and maintenance therapy with olaparib. Testing for MSI/MMR deficiency is recommended to identify patients who are candidates to receive immunotherapy. Presence of these germline mu-tations has also helped recognize unaffected indi-viduals who might be at high risk for PDAC and may benefit from screening. With the increasing use of multigene panels, further research is needed to understand the clinical relevance of new genes being identified and incorporating them in targeted therapy.

CLINICS CARE POINTS

- Pearls: *BRCA1 (2.4% to 0.35%) /BRCA2 (5.2% to 1.34%) are the most frequently identified germline mutations in PDAC patients.*

- Pitfalls: Multigene panels can identify patho-genic variants for which clinical management is unclear due to limited data on cancer risk and often are not targettable.

- Pearls: PARP Inhibitors can be used to target patients with PDAC and germline mutations in DNA repair genes.

- Pearls: PDAC screening is reccomended for asymptomatic individuals harbouring germ-line mutations.

ACKNOWLEDGMENTS

This study was supported by grants to F. McAllister from the NCI (1R37CA237384–01A1), CPRIT (RP200173), V Foundation Translational Award, Andrew Sabin Family Fellowship, SU2C-Lustgarten Foundation Pancreatic Cancer Interception Translational Cancer Research Grant (Grant Number: SU2C-AACR-DT25-17).and philanthropic support from the MD Anderson Moonshot Programs. A. Maitra is supported by the Khalifa Bin Zayed Al-Nahyan Foundation and P50CA221707.

DISCLOSURE

A. Maitra receives royalties for a pancreatic cancer biomarker test from Cosmos Wisdom Biotechnology, and this financial relationship is managed and monitored by the UTMDACC Conflict of Interest Committee. A. Maitra is also listed as an inventor on a patent that has been licensed by Johns Hopkins University to Thrive Earlier Detection. A. Maitra is a consultant for Freenome and Tezcat Biotechnology. F. McAllister is an SAB Member at Neologics Bio.M.B. Yurgelun receives research funding from Janssen Pharmaceuticals.

REFERENCES

1. Siegel RL, Miller KD, Fuchs HE, et al. Cancer statistics, 2022. CA Cancer J Clin 2022;72(1):7–33.
2. Stoffel EM, McKernin SE, Brand R, et al. Evaluating susceptibility to pancreatic cancer: ASCO provisional clinical opinion. J Clin Oncol 2019;37(2): 153–64.
3. Brand R, Borazanci E, Speare V, et al. Prospective study of germline genetic testing in incident cases of pancreatic adenocarcinoma. Cancer 2018; 124(17):3520–7.
4. Dudley B, Karloski E, Monzon FA, et al. Germline mutation prevalence in individuals with pancreatic cancer and a history of previous malignancy. Cancer 2018;124(8):1691–700.
5. Grant RC, Selander I, Connor AA, et al. Prevalence of germline mutations in cancer predisposition genes in patients with pancreatic cancer. Gastroenterology 2015;148(3):556–64.
6. Hu C, Hart SN, Polley EC, et al. Association between inherited germline mutations in cancer predisposition genes and risk of pancreatic cancer. Jama 2018;319(23):2401–9.
7. Lowery MA, Wong W, Jordan EJ, et al. Prospective evaluation of germline alterations in patients with exocrine pancreatic neoplasms. JNCI: J Natl Cancer Inst 2018;110(10):1067–74.
8. McKay S, Humphris J, Johns A, et al. Abstract A02: assessment of germline cancer predisposition genes in 392 unselected pancreatic cancer patients. Philadelphia, PA: AACR; 2016.
9. Yurgelun MB, Chittenden AB, Morales-Oyarvide V, et al. Germline cancer susceptibility gene variants, somatic second hits, and survival outcomes in patients with resected pancreatic cancer. Genet Med 2019;21(1):213–23.
10. Goldstein JB, Zhao L, Wang X, et al. Germline DNA sequencing reveals novel mutations predictive of overall survival in a cohort of patients with pancreatic cancer. Clin Cancer Res 2020;26(6): 1385–94.
11. Bannon SA, Montiel MF, Goldstein JB, et al. High prevalence of hereditary cancer syndromes and outcomes in adults with early-onset pancreatic cancer. Cancer Prev Res 2018;11(11):679–86.
12. Shindo K, Yu J, Suenaga M, et al. Deleterious germline mutations in patients with apparently sporadic pancreatic adenocarcinoma. J Clin Oncol 2017; 35(30):3382.
13. NCCN Guidelines NCCN. Pancreatic Adenocarcinoma, Version 2.2021. webpage 2021.
14. Pishvaian MJ, Blais EM, Brody JR, et al. Overall survival in patients with pancreatic cancer receiving matched therapies following molecular profiling: a retrospective analysis of the Know Your Tumor registry trial. Lancet Oncol 2020;21(4):508–18.
15. Golan T, Hammel P, Reni M, et al. Maintenance olaparib for germline BRCA-mutated metastatic pancreatic cancer. N Engl J Med 2019;381(4): 317–27.
16. FDA. FDA approves olaparib for gBRCAm metastatic pancreatic adenocarcinoma. 2019.
17. Lowery MA, Kelsen DP, Capanu M, et al. Phase II trial of veliparib in patients with previously treated BRCA-mutated pancreas ductal adenocarcinoma. Eur J Cancer 2018;89:19–26.
18. Shroff RT, Hendifar A, McWilliams RR, et al. Rucaparib monotherapy in patients with pancreatic cancer and a known deleterious BRCA mutation. JCO precision Oncol 2018;2:1–15.
19. FDA. FDA grants accelerated approval to pembrolizumab for first tissue/site agnostic indication. 2017.
20. Hester R, Mazur PK, McAllister F. Immunotherapy in Pancreatic Adenocarcinoma: Beyond "Copy/Paste". Clin Cancer Res 2021;27(23):6287–97.
21. Royal RE, Levy C, Turner K, et al. Phase 2 trial of single agent Ipilimumab (anti-CTLA-4) for locally advanced or metastatic pancreatic adenocarcinoma. J Immunother 2010;33(8):828.
22. O'Reilly EM, Oh D-Y, Dhani N, et al. Durvalumab with or without tremelimumab for patients with metastatic pancreatic ductal adenocarcinoma: a phase 2 randomized clinical trial. JAMA Oncol 2019;5(10): 1431–8.

23. Aglietta M, Barone C, Sawyer M, et al. A phase I dose escalation trial of tremelimumab (CP-675,206) in combination with gemcitabine in chemotherapy-naive patients with metastatic pancreatic cancer. Ann Oncol 2014;25(9):1750–5.

24. Weiss GJ, Blaydorn L, Beck J, et al. Phase Ib/II study of gemcitabine, nab-paclitaxel, and pembrolizumab in metastatic pancreatic adenocarcinoma. Invest New Drugs 2018;36(1):96–102.

25. Parikh AR, Szabolcs A, Allen JN, et al. Radiation therapy enhances immunotherapy response in microsatellite stable colorectal and pancreatic adenocarcinoma in a phase II trial. Nat Cancer 2021; 2(11):1124–35.

26. Daly MB, Pal T, Berry MP, et al. Genetic/familial high-risk assessment: breast, ovarian, and pancreatic, version 2.2021, NCCN clinical practice guidelines in oncology. J Natl Compr Cancer Netw 2021; 19(1):77–102.

27. Furniss CS, Yurgelun MB, Ukaegbu C, et al. Novel Models of Genetic Education and Testing for Pancreatic Cancer Interception: Preliminary Results from the GENERATE Study. Cancer Prev Res 2021; 14(11):1021–32.

28. Salo-Mullen EE, O'Reilly EM, Kelsen DP, et al. Identification of germline genetic mutations in patients with pancreatic cancer. Cancer 2015;121(24): 4382–8.

29. Vasen H, Ibrahim I, Ponce CG, et al. Benefit of surveillance for pancreatic cancer in high-risk individuals: outcome of long-term prospective follow-up studies from three European expert centers. J Clin Oncol 2016;34(17):2010.

30. Konings I, Canto MI, Almario J, et al. Surveillance for pancreatic cancer in high-risk individuals. BJS open 2019;3(5):656–65.

31. Canto MI, Almario JA, Schulick RD, et al. Risk of neoplastic progression in individuals at high risk for pancreatic cancer undergoing long-term surveillance. Gastroenterology 2018;155(3):740–51.e2.

32. Goggins M, Schutte M, Lu J, et al. Germline BRCA2 gene mutations in patients with apparently sporadic pancreatic carcinomas. Cancer Res 1996;56(23): 5360–4.

33. Friedenson B. BRCA1 and BRCA2 pathways and the risk of cancers other than breast or ovarian. Medscape Gen Med 2005;7(2):60.

34. Lynch HT, Deters CA, Snyder CL, et al. BRCA1 and pancreatic cancer: pedigree findings and their causal relationships. Cancer Genet Cytogenet 2005;158(2):119–25.

35. Couch FJ, Johnson MR, Rabe KG, et al. The prevalence of BRCA2 mutations in familial pancreatic cancer. Cancer Epidemiol Prev Biomarkers 2007;16(2):342–6.

36. Hahn SA, Greenhalf B, Ellis I, et al. BRCA2 germline mutations in familial pancreatic carcinoma. J Natl Cancer Inst 2003;95(3):214–21.

37. Murphy KM, Brune KA, Griffin C, et al. Evaluation of candidate genes MAP2K4, MADH4, ACVR1B, and BRCA2 in familial pancreatic cancer: deleterious BRCA2 mutations in 17. Cancer Res 2002;62(13): 3789–93.

38. Hu C, Hart SN, Bamlet WR, et al. Prevalence of pathogenic mutations in cancer predisposition genes among pancreatic cancer patients. Cancer Epidemiol Prev Biomarkers 2016;25(1):207–11.

39. Jones S, Hruban RH, Kamiyama M, et al. Exomic sequencing identifies PALB2 as a pancreatic cancer susceptibility gene. Science 2009;324(5924): 217.

40. Hofstatter EW, Domchek SM, Miron A, et al. PALB2 mutations in familial breast and pancreatic cancer. Fam Cancer 2011;10(2):225–31.

41. Borecka M, Zemankova P, Vocka M, et al. Mutation analysis of the PALB2 gene in unselected pancreatic cancer patients in the Czech Republic. Cancer Genet 2016;209(5):199–204.

42. Nanda N, Roberts NJ. ATM serine/threonine kinase and its role in pancreatic risk. Genes 2020;11(1): 108.

43. Roberts NJ, Jiao Y, Yu J, et al. ATM mutations in hereditary pancreatic cancer patients. Cancer Discov 2012;2(1):41.

44. Skaro M, Nanda N, Gauthier C, et al. Prevalence of germline mutations associated with cancer risk in patients with intraductal papillary mucinous neoplasms. Gastroenterology 2019;156(6):1905–13.

45. Vilar E, Gruber SB. Microsatellite instability in colorectal cancer—the stable evidence. Nat Rev Clin Oncol 2010;7(3):153–62.

46. Bujanda L, Herreros-Villanueva M. Pancreatic cancer in lynch syndrome patients. J Cancer 2017; 8(18):3667.

47. Kastrinos F, Mukherjee B, Tayob N, et al. Risk of pancreatic cancer in families with Lynch syndrome. Jama 2009;302(16):1790–5.

48. Hu ZI, Shia J, Stadler ZK, et al. Evaluating mismatch repair deficiency in pancreatic adenocarcinoma: challenges and recommendations. Clin Cancer Res 2018;24(6):1326–36.

49. Macherla S, Laks S, Naqash AR, et al. Emerging role of immune checkpoint blockade in pancreatic cancer. Int J Mol Sci 2018;19(11):3505.

50. McWilliams RR, Wieben ED, Rabe KG, et al. Prevalence of CDKN2A mutations in pancreatic cancer patients: implications for genetic counseling. Eur J Hum Genet 2011;19(4):472–8.

51. Ibrahim IS, Brückner C, Carrato A, et al. Incidental findings in pancreas screening programs for high-risk individuals: Results from three European expert centers. United Eur Gastroenterol J 2019;7(5):682–8.

52. Sahin F, Maitra A, Argani P, et al. Loss of Stk11/Lkb1 expression in pancreatic and biliary neoplasms. Mod Pathol 2003;16(7):686–91.

53. Hezel A, Bardeesy N. LKB1; linking cell structure and tumor suppression. Oncogene 2008;27(55): 6908–19.

54. Guldberg P, Ahrenkiel V, Seremet T, et al. Somatic mutation of the Peutz-Jeghers syndrome gene, LKB1/STK11, in malignant melanoma. Oncogene 1999;18(9):1777–80.

55. Beggs A, Latchford AR, Vasen HF, et al. Peutz–Jeghers syndrome: a systematic review and recommendations for management. Gut 2010;59(7): 975–86.

56. Resta N, Pierannunzio D, Lenato GM, et al. Cancer risk associated with STK11/LKB1 germline mutations in Peutz–Jeghers syndrome patients: Results of an Italian multicenter study. Dig Liver Dis 2013; 45(7):606–11.

57. Mork M, Quesada PR, Bannon S, et al. Pancreatic cancer early detection and interception in an atypical case of Peutz-Jeghers syndrome. Pancreas 2019;48(4):e29.

58. Cazacu IM, Farkas N, Garami A, et al. Pancreatitis-associated genes and pancreatic cancer risk: a systematic review and meta-analysis. Pancreas 2018; 47(9):1078.

59. Shelton CA, Umapathy C, Stello K, et al. Hereditary pancreatitis in the United States: survival and rates of pancreatic cancer. Am J Gastroenterol 2018; 113(9):1376.

60. Howes N, Lerch MM, Greenhalf W, et al. Clinical and genetic characteristics of hereditary pancreatitis in Europe. Clin Gastroenterol Hepatol 2004;2(3): 252–61.

61. Matsubayashi H, Fukushima N, Sato N, et al. Polymorphisms of SPINK1 N34S and CFTR in patients with sporadic and familial pancreatic cancer. Cancer Biol Ther 2003;2(6):652–5.

62. Shindo K, Yu J, Suenaga M, et al. Lack of association between the pancreatitis risk allele CEL-HYB and pancreatic cancer. Oncotarget 2017;8(31): 50824.

63. Pereira F, Teixeira MR, Ribeiro MD, et al. Multi-Gene Panel Testing in Gastroenterology: Are We Ready for the Results? GE-Portuguese J Gastroenterol 2021; 28(6):403–9.

64. Okur V, Chung WK. The impact of hereditary cancer gene panels on clinical care and lessons learned. Mol Case Stud 2017;3(6):a002154.

65. Green RC, Berg JS, Grody WW, et al. ACMG recommendations for reporting of incidental findings in clinical exome and genome sequencing. Genet Med 2013;15(7):565–74.

66. Mandelker D, Zhang L, Kemel Y, et al. Mutation detection in patients with advanced cancer by universal sequencing of cancer-related genes in tumor and normal DNA vs guideline-based germline testing. Jama 2017;318(9):825–35.

67. NCCN. NCCN Guidelines Version 2.2021 Genetic/Familial High-Risk Assessment: Breast, Ovarian, and Pancreatic. 2021.

68. Fountzilas C, Kaklamani VG. Multi-Gene panel testing in breast cancer management. Cham, Switzerland: Optimizing Breast Cancer Management; 2018. p. 121–40.

69. Kurian AW, Ford JM. Multigene panel testing in oncology practice: how should we respond? JAMA Oncol 2015;1(3):277–8.

70. Golan T, Sella T, O'Reilly EM, et al. Overall survival and clinical characteristics of BRCA mutation carriers with stage I/II pancreatic cancer. Br J Cancer 2017;116(6):697–702.

71. Pokataev I, Fedyanin M, Polyanskaya E, et al. Efficacy of platinum-based chemotherapy and prognosis of patients with pancreatic cancer with homologous recombination deficiency: comparative analysis of published clinical studies. ESMO open 2020;5(1):e000578.

72. Perkhofer L, Gout J, Roger E, et al. DNA damage repair as a target in pancreatic cancer: state-of-the-art and future perspectives. Gut 2021;70(3): 606–17.

73. O'Reilly EM, Lee JW, Zalupski M, et al. Randomized, multicenter, phase II trial of gemcitabine and cisplatin with or without veliparib in patients with pancreas adenocarcinoma and a germline BRCA/PALB2 mutation. J Clin Oncol 2020;38(13): 1378.

74. Kaufman B, Shapira-Frommer R, Schmutzler RK, et al. Olaparib monotherapy in patients with advanced cancer and a germline BRCA1/2 mutation. J Clin Oncol 2015;33(3):244.

75. Min A, Im S-A, Yoon Y-K, et al. RAD51C-deficient cancer cells are highly sensitive to the PARP inhibitor olaparib. Mol Cancer Ther 2013;12(6):865–77.

76. A Randomized Study of Olaparib or Placebo in Patients With Surgically Removed Pancreatic Cancer Who Have a BRCA1, BRCA2 or PALB2 Mutation, The APOLLO Trial.

77. Armstrong SA, Schultz CW, Azimi-Sadjadi A, et al. ATM dysfunction in pancreatic adenocarcinoma and associated therapeutic implications. Mol Cancer Ther 2019;18(11):1899–908.

78. Javle M, Shacham-Shmueli E, Xiao L, et al. Olaparib monotherapy for previously treated pancreatic cancer with DNA damage repair genetic alterations other than germline BRCA variants: findings from 2 phase 2 nonrandomized clinical trials. JAMA Oncol 2021;7(5):693–9.

79. Ayars M, Eshleman J, Goggins M. Susceptibility of ATM-deficient pancreatic cancer cells to radiation. Cell Cycle 2017;16(10):991–8.

80. Zhang Q, Green MD, Lang X, et al. Inhibition of ATM increases interferon signaling and sensitizes

pancreatic cancer to immune checkpoint blockade therapy. Cancer Res 2019;79(15):3940–51.

81. Testing the Addition of an Anti-cancer Drug, BAY 1895344 ATR Inhibitor, to the Chemotherapy Treatment (Gemcitabine) for Advanced Pancreatic and Ovarian Cancer, and Advanced Solid Tumors.

82. Chu QS, Jonker DJ, Provencher DM, et al. A phase Ib study of oral Chk1 inhibitor LY2880070 in combination with gemcitabine in patients with advanced or metastatic cancer. Alexandria, VA: American Society of Clinical Oncology; 2020.

83. Dose Escalation Trial of AZD1775 and Gemcitabine (+Radiation) for Unresectable Adenocarcinoma of the Pancreas.

84. Lemery S, Keegan P, Pazdur R. First FDA approval agnostic of cancer site-when a biomarker defines the indication. N Engl J Med 2017;377(15):1409–12.

85. Marabelle A, Le DT, Ascierto PA, et al. Efficacy of pembrolizumab in patients with noncolorectal high microsatellite instability/mismatch repair–deficient cancer: Results from the phase II KEYNOTE-158 study. J Clin Oncol 2020;38(1):1.

86. Study of Pembrolizumab (MK-3475) in Participants With Advanced Solid Tumors (MK-3475-158/KEYNOTE-158).

87. A Study of XmAb®22841 Monotherapy & in Combination w/Pembrolizumab in Subjects w/Selected Advanced Solid Tumors.

88. Sonidegib and Pembrolizumab in Treating Patients With Advanced Solid Tumors.

89. Pembrolizumab In Combination With Debio 1143 In Pancreatic and Colorectal Advanced/Metastatic Adenocarcinoma.

90. Kalyan A, Kircher SM, Mohindra NA, et al. Ipilimumab and gemcitabine for advanced pancreas cancer: a phase Ib study. Alexandria, VA: American Society of Clinical Oncology; 2016.

91. Mohindra NA, Kircher SM, Nimeiri HS, et al. Results of the phase Ib study of ipilimumab and gemcitabine for advanced pancreas cancer. American Society of Clinical Oncology; 2015.

92. Lucas AL, Kastrinos F. Screening for pancreatic cancer. Jama 2019;322(5):407–8.

93. Network NCC. NCCN guidelines version 1.2022 pancreatic cancer screening. 2022. Available at: https://www.nccn.org/professionals/physician_gls/pdf/genetics_bop.pdf. Accessed March 6, 2022.

94. Overbeek KA, Levink IJ, Koopmann BD, et al. Long-term yield of pancreatic cancer surveillance in high-risk individuals. Gut 2022;71(6):1152–60.

95. Yurgelun MB, Ukaegbu CI, Furniss CS, et al. Improving cascade genetic testing for families with inherited pancreatic cancer (PDAC) risk: the GENetic Education, Risk Assessment and TEsting (GENERATE) study. Alexandria, VA: American Society of Clinical Oncology; 2020.

APPENDIX

Supplementary Table 1
Germline prevalence across study groups with an unselected population along with number of genes tested

Sno.	Study Name	Percentage	No of Genes Tested (n)	Genes Detected (n)	Germline Prevalence (n)	Total Patients (n)
1	McWilliams Robert R., et al.	0.58%	1	1	9	1537
2	Shindo, Koji, et al.	3.90%	32	7	33	854
3	Holter, Spring, et al.	4.50%	2	2	14	306
4	Özcelik, Hilmi, et al.	4.80%	1	1	2	41
5	McKay, Skye, et al.	5.90%	13	7	23	392
6	Bannon et al.	6.81%	13	5	9	132
7	Goggins, Michael, et al.	7.30%	1	1	3	41
8	Hu, Chunling, et al.	8.20%	21	19	249	3030
9	Yurgelun, Matthew B., et al.	9.70%	24	14	28	289
10	Brand, Randall, et al.	9.70%	32	10	29	298
11	Goldstein et al.	19.50%	263	16	26	133
12	Lowery, Maeve A., et al.	19.80%	76	24	122	615

Supplementary Table 2
Individual germline mutation prevalence of the commonly identified genes across various study cohorts

Study Groups	ATM	BRCA1	BRCA2	CDKN2A	CHEK2	MLH1	MSH2	MSH6	PALB2	PMS2	TP53
Yurgelun, Matthew B., et al.	1.38%	1.03%	1.38%	0.69%	1.03%		0.34%	0.69%	0.34%		0.34%
Holter, Spring, et al.		0.98%	3.59%								
Goggins, Michael, et al.			7.31%								
Hu, Chunling, et al.	2.27%	0.59%	1.94%	0.33%	1.08%	0.16%	0.03%	0.23%	0.39%	0.06%	0.19%
Shindo, Koji, et al.	1.17%	0.35%	1.40%	0.11%		0.23%		0.23%			0.11%
Banon et al.	2.27%	1.15%	1.15%	0.75%							0.75%
Brand, Randall, et al.	3.35%	1.34%	1.34%	0.33%	1.67%		0.33%	0.33%	0.33%		0.33%
McWilliams, Robert R., et al.				0.58%							
Özcelik, Hilmi, et al.			4.87%								
McKay, Skye, et al.	1.02%	0.76%	2.29%	0.51%				0.76%	0.25%		
Goldstein et al.	2.25%	1.50%	1.50%	0.75%	3.00%			0.75%			0.75%
Lowery, Maeve A., et al.	1.78%	2.40%	5.70%	0.97%	3.08%	0.16%	0.16%	0.16%	0.16%	0.48%	0.16%
Mean	1.94%	1.16%	2.89%	0.56%	1.97%	0.18%	0.18%	0.35%	0.42%	0.28%	0.37%

Total Pancreatectomy with Islet Autotransplantation
New Insights on the Pathology and Pathogenesis of Chronic Pancreatitis from Tissue Research

Sadé M.B. Finn, MD[a], Melena D. Bellin, MD, MS[b],*

KEYWORDS

• Total pancreatectomy • Pancreatitis • TPIAT • Chronic pancreatitis • Hereditary pancreatitis

Key points

- A new consensus definition of chronic pancreatitis (CP) is a pathologic fibroinflammatory syndrome of the pancreas in individuals with genetic, environmental, and/or other risk factors who develop persistent pathologic responses to parenchymal injury or stress.
- Distinct immune subpopulation-mediated mechanisms may underlie the pathogenesis of hereditary and idiopathic CP.
- Histopathology is not routinely used for the clinical diagnosis of CP. Cardinal clinical features of CP along with radiographic imaging findings, and histopathology if available, are used to diagnosis CP.

ABSTRACT

Total pancreatectomy with islet autotransplantation (TPIAT) is a surgical procedure undertaken in some patients with severe pain or disability from recurrent acute and chronic pancreatitis (CP). TPIAT provides a rare opportunity to study human pancreas tissue from patients affected with pancreatitis, and particularly from patients with genetic forms of pancreatitis. Research to date suggests distinct histopathology and potentially differential pathophysiology of distinct etiologies of CP. Histopathology specimens have helped better define the success and limitations of clinical diagnostic imaging tools, such as magnetic retrograde cholangiopancreatography and endoscopic ultrasound.

INTRODUCTION

Chronic pancreatitis (CP) has classically been defined as a syndrome of chronic progressive pancreatic inflammation leading to atrophy and fibrosis of the pancreas and resulting in exocrine and endocrine dysfunction.[1,2] However, this definition proves problematic in its focus on advanced stages of CP. Recently, a new consensus mechanism-based definition of CP was put forth, describing CP as a pathologic fibroinflammatory syndrome of the pancreas in an individual with genetic, environmental, and/or other risk factors who develops persistent pathologic responses to parenchymal injury or stress, which may include features of pancreatic atrophy, fibrosis, pain syndromes, ductal distortion and strictures,

a Department of Surgery, University of Minnesota Medical School, 420 Delaware Street Southeast, Minneapolis, MN 55455, USA; b Department of Pediatrics and Department of Surgery, University of Minnesota Medical School, MMC 391, 420 Delaware Street Southeast, Minneapolis, MN 55455, USA
* Corresponding author.
E-mail address: bell0130@umn.edu

Surgical Pathology 15 (2022) 503–509
https://doi.org/10.1016/j.path.2022.05.005
1875-9181/22/© 2022 Elsevier Inc. All rights reserved.

surgpath.theclinics.com

calcifications, and pancreatic endocrine and/or exocrine dysfunction.[2] Total pancreatectomy with islet autotransplantation (TPIAT) is a surgical treatment indicated for select patients with recurrent acute pancreatitis or CP who suffer from debilitating pain refractory to medical and endoscopic therapies. In this review, we will highlight recent advancements in our understanding of the pathogenesis of CP and in noninvasive tools for the diagnosis of CP because of pancreatic specimen availability due to TPIAT.

TOTAL PANCREATECTOMY WITH ISLET AUTOTRANSPLANTATION

In the evolution to CP, many (but not all) individuals present first with recurrent acute pancreatitis, with progression to clear CP on imaging coinciding with clinical progression of the disease.[3] Defining the point at which the disease becomes "chronic" remains a challenge; when patients with recurrent acute pancreatitis undergo TPIAT, the majority has mild or patchy fibrosis on histopathology consistent with early CP at the time of pancreas resection.[4] There is no curative therapy for CP and management primarily focuses on treating symptoms and complications of the disease. Initial therapies may include analgesics, fluid therapy, antioxidants, or pancreatic enzyme therapy.[5,6] Patients with ductal stones or strictures may benefit from endoscopic retrograde cholangiopancreatography (ERCP).[7] When disease is disabling despite adequate medical and endoscopic therapy, surgical therapies may be considered.

One surgical approach to treat CP is TPIAT. In this procedure, the entire pancreas is removed to eliminate the generator of the pain, and the islets are isolated and transplanted intraportally into the liver to prevent or minimize the severity of postsurgical diabetes.[8] In brief, TPIAT is performed at our institution as a pylorus-preserving total pancreatectomy with ligation of the pancreatic vascular just before removal followed by Roux-en-Y duodenojejunostomy reconstruction. Excisional biopsies from the pancreatic head, body, and/or tail are collected for histologic analysis. The pancreatic tissue is then enzymatically disrupted using injection of intraductal collagenase and neutral protease solutions, followed by mechanical disruption use the semiautomated method of Ricordi.[9]

Because TPIAT is a major surgical procedure with long-term health risks, candidates must be carefully evaluated for appropriateness for TPIAT. The most important first step is to confirm the diagnosis of recurrent acute or CP as the cause of the abdominal pain. According to the International Consensus Guidelines, candidates for TPIAT should have documented chronic narcotic dependence or impaired quality of life, have an irreversible cause of CP, have symptoms unresponsive to maximal medical and endoscopic therapies, have ongoing abdominal pain requiring routine narcotics for CP, and have adequate islet function.[1,10] In particular, TPIAT has been increasingly used for patients with small duct disease, where traditional surgical drainage procedures are not an option, and in children and young adults with genetic forms of pancreatitis.[11,12]

Multiple institutions performing TPIAT have reported successful reduction of pain, reduced opioid use, and overall improved quality of life as measured by standardized questionnaires at 1 to 5 years after TPIAT.[13–15] In our experience, about 85% of patients report reduced or resolved pain, whereas 15% report the same level of pain despite pancreatic resection.[14] Insulin independence rates vary but, in general, around 1 in every 3 to 4 patients undergoing TPIAT becomes completely insulin independent, and most individuals on insulin demonstrate partial function of the islet graft by measurable circulating C-peptide.[14,15] In a cohort of 215 pediatric and adult patients more than 10 years out from TPIAT, approximately 77% were insulin-independent or had partial graft function and 6% reported pancreatitis-type pain at 1 year after TPIAT, whereas 47% were insulin-independent or had partial graft function and 18% reported pancreatitis-type pain at 10 years after TPIAT, demonstrating the durability of TPIAT for the treatment of CP-related abdominal pain.[10]

CP can affect the structural and functional integrity of the pancreas in a heterogenous manner both grossly and histologically, depending on the duration of disease and the cause of CP.[2,16,17] TPIAT offers the unique opportunity to study pancreatic specimens from affected patients, often before very late stage complications of CP such as diabetes have developed. Patients undergoing TPIAT are enriched particularly for genetic risk factors and idiopathic disease, allowing novel investigations into tissue histology and disease pathophysiology with the most common causes of CP: alcoholic, hereditary, and idiopathic.

EARLY OBSERVATIONS AND THEORIES ON THE PATHOPHYSIOLOGY OF CHRONIC PANCREATITIS USING TISSUE SPECIMENS

Several risk factors for CP have been identified including chronic heavy alcohol abuse, gene mutations, smoking, autoimmune syndromes, metabolic disturbances, toxic factors, or anatomic abnormalities. Regardless of the cause, the underlying pathogenesis of CP results from recurrent acute pancreatitis instigating injury and fibrotic remodeling of the pancreas. In 2007, Kloppel summarized the main histologic findings of various causes of CP from cadavers and/or tumor-related pancreatic resections.[17] He reported uneven distribution of fibrosis and associated ductal dilation in alcoholic CP. Intralobular ducts are often filled with protein plugs that progress to calculi as the disease becomes more advanced. Several hypotheses were proposed based on these tissue findings to explain the pathogenesis of alcoholic CP. The plug hypothesis suggested that chronic alcohol consumption increases pancreatic protein concentration with subsequent precipitation of plug-forming secretions in the ducts that later calcify. An alternate theory termed the necrosis-fibrosis hypothesis proposed that the resorption of large areas of fat necrosis and hemorrhagic necrosis during acute pancreatitis induce fibrosis, explaining the perilobular fibrosis pattern. During the more recent decade, pancreatic stellate cells have been identified as a major player in the genesis of pancreatic fibrosis.[18]

DECIPHERING UNIQUE PATHWAYS BASED ON THE CAUSE OF CHRONIC PANCREATITIS

Although heavy alcohol consumption is a common risk factor for CP, patients with alcohol abuse are often not suitable candidates for TPIAT due to other medical comorbidities such as liver disease or ongoing substance use. Thus, histologic studies with large contributions from patients with alcoholic CP undergoing TPIAT are limited. RNA sequencing data from a small cohort of alcoholic CP undergoing TPIAT found enriched pathways involved in ion transport and binding, providing a foundation for additional studies to investigate molecular pathogenesis of alcoholic CP.[19]

Recent studies of pancreatic tissue from patients undergoing TPIAT have yielded insight into immunohistologic differences between hereditary and idiopathic CP. In a study of 40 patients undergoing TPIAT for hereditary CP (n = 27) and for idiopathic CP (n = 13), Lee and colleagues[20] found a striking pattern of macrophage predominant infiltration of the pancreas in idiopathic disease versus T-cell infiltrates in hereditary CP. Specifically, a significant expansion of anti-inflammatory CD68$^+$CD11c$^-$ (M2) macrophage cells, M2 macrophage cytokines (interleukin [IL]-4, IL-13) and expression of innate (IL-21, IL-23) and Th2 (IL-5, IL-9, and IL-31) cytokine levels were observed in idiopathic CP pancreatic tissue compared with hereditary CP pancreatic

tissue. Conversely, pancreatic tissues from patients with hereditary CP had significantly dominant subpopulations of CD3$^+$CD4$^+$ helper T cells compared with idiopathic CP, suggesting distinct immune mechanisms underlying the different causes.[20] A separate study of RNA sequencing and sequence data enrichment using archived frozen pancreatic biopsy samples taken from patients with hereditary CP (n = 6) and idiopathic CP (n = 8) suggested significantly more tissue regeneration and repair in hereditary CP as evidenced by upregulated genes in pathways involved in tissue remodeling, cell proliferation, development, and MMP12 gene compared with pancreatic tissue from individuals with idiopathic CP.[19] These studies exemplify opportunities to use fresh tissue or specially stored specimens (for RNASeq) in pancreatitis research.

Other studies have used conventional paraffin-embedded stored samples for histopathological analyses in specific genetic forms of CP. Histologic findings from serine protease 1 (PRSS1)-related CP support a sequential pattern of lipomatous pancreatic atrophy (Fig. 1). In a cohort study of 10 patients aged 6 to 68 years with heterozygous PRSS1 germline mutation undergoing TPIAT (n = 6) or total pancreatectomy for malignancy (n = 4), Singhi and colleagues[21] found PRSS1 to be associated with patchy parenchymal loss with replacement by loosely packed, perilobular and interlobular fibrosis in specimens from pediatric patients. Pancreatic specimens from young adults aged 28 to 30 years were similar to pediatric specimens but also showed intermingled adipocytes and ductal alterations, including ectasia, squamous metaplasia, and intraductal calcifications. Fatty replacement and localized fibrosis seemed to be progressive findings as patients with PRSS1 aged. Among the study's oldest patients, the pancreas was consistently soft and markedly atrophied, with histologic findings of pancreatic parenchyma almost entirely replaced by mature adipose tissue, scattered islets of Langerhans, and fibrosis primarily periductal and cuffing dilated main pancreatic and larger interlobular ducts that contained intraductal calcifications.[21]

Unlike PRSS1-related CP, serine peptidase inhibitor Kazal type 1 (SPINK1)-related CP demonstrates progressive loss of acinar cell and ductal epithelium with extensive parenchymal fibrosis. In a cohort study of 28 patients aged 5 to 48 years with germline mutation in SPINK1 undergoing TPIAT for chronic pain, Singhi and colleagues[22] reported histologic findings in pancreatic specimens based on duration of abdominal pain at the time of TPIAT. Multifocal, cytoplasmic vacuolization of acinar parenchyma with mild intralobular fibrosis was observed in specimens from patients reporting

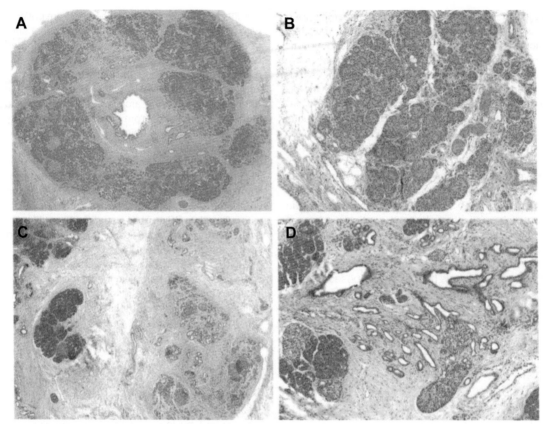

Fig. 1. A sequential pattern of histologic changes identified in patients with germline mutations in PRSS1. (*A*) Pancreata from pediatric patients were characterized by patchy parenchymal loss with replacement by loosely packed, perilobular and interlobular fibrosis. In addition, a mild increase in chronic inflammation was identified and primarily localized around dilated pancreatic ducts. (*B*) At the periphery of the pancreas, a greater loss of acinar and ductal tissue was seen with residual islet of Langerhans organized in aggregates and surrounded by mature adipocytes and thin wisps of collagen. (*C*) In young adults, progressive parenchymal collapse was observed with replacement by perilobular and interlobular fibrosis and scattered adipocytes. (*D*) Ductal alterations including ectasia and metaplasia were common findings. (Trikudanathan, Guru MD et al., FACG1 Diagnostic Performance of Contrast-Enhanced MRI With Secretin-Stimulated MRCP for Non-Calcific Chronic Pancreatitis: A Comparison With Histopathology, American Journal of Gastroenterology: November 2015 - Volume 110 - Issue 11 - p 1598–1606, https://doi.org/10.1038/ajg.2015.297.)

less than 4 years of abdominal pain (n = 10). If patients were cocarriers of CFTR mutations, focal intralobular and extralobular lipomatous infiltrates were also present. Progressive loss of acinar parenchyma and thick bundles of collagen, fibroblasts, and scattered islands of neutrophilic inflammation contributing to mild interlobular, intralobular, and perilobular fibrosis was observed in SPINK1 patients (n = 6) who reported abdominal pain for 4 to 7 years. With abdominal pain duration of 7 to 15 years (n = 8), ductal ectasia, squamous metaplasia, and intraductal concretions were reported in addition to acinar cell epithelium loss. Near-complete to complete loss of acinar and ductal epithelium and extensive/severe parenchymal fibrosis with residual islets of Langerhans embedded in fibrosis was seen in specimens from

patients reporting abdominal pain between 21 and 25 years (n = 4). Unlike PRSS1, the progressive loss of primarily exocrine parenchyma and replacement by prominent fibrosis seen in SPINK1 seems age-independent and associated with the duration of reported abdominal pain.

ADVANCEMENTS IN DIAGNOSIS OF CHRONIC PANCREATITIS, GUIDED BY ACCESS TO HISTOPATHOLOGY

Histopathology alone is not routinely used for the clinical diagnosis of CP due to the invasive nature and safety risk associated with pancreatic biopsy. Although tissue offers advantages over clinical imaging studies, the use of histopathology still carries significant limitations as a diagnostic test due to the lack of a reproducible and universally accepted histologic grading system.[16] Scoring systems for the extent of fibrosis, such as the often-used fibrosis scoring system proposed by Kloppel and Maillet or its later iteration that accounts for pancreatic function by Ammann and colleagues, are not validated for clinical use. Furthermore, the fibrosis scoring systems that are used in research are only valid for advanced CP because access to pancreatic specimens from individuals with suspected early CP is rare. It is acknowledged that the cardinal features of CP are the triad of fibrosis, loss of acinar tissue, and ductal changes (Fig. 2). However, there is no consensus among pathologists about what minimum features are required to make the diagnosis of CP or how to grade the features.[16] TPIAT offers an opportunity to develop this field, as patients undergo TPIAT at differing stages of disease, from recurrent AP with minimal fibrosis to advanced CP.

The determination of CP is multidisciplinary. According to the International Consensus Guidelines for CP, histopathology is presently not the gold standard for the diagnosis of CP, and the pathologist should also consider the clinical history and radiologic features of the pancreas in making the diagnosis.[16] The diagnosis of longstanding, advanced calcific CP with traditional cross-sectional imaging is relatively straightforward. Computed tomography is highly sensitive for advanced CP with calcifications, atrophy, fat replacement, and ductal dilation.[23] Accurate diagnosis of noncalcific CP in patients presenting with chronic abdominal pain is challenging because surgical histopathology is often unavailable until the disease is advanced, refractor to other therapies, or associated with metaplasia or malignancy. Presently, endoscopic ultrasound (EUS) and magnetic resonance imaging (MRI) with or without secretin-stimulated magnetic

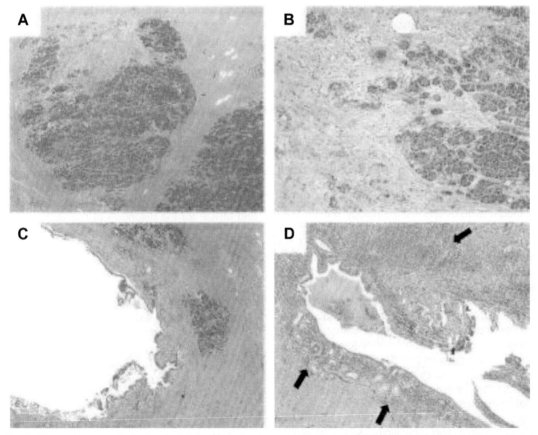

Fig. 2. Cardinal histopathological features of nonautoimmune CP. A triad of (A) (H&E, 25×) interlobular and intralobular collagen-rich fibrosis, (B) (H&E, 100×) atrophy of acinar parenchyma, and duct changes such as (C) (H&E, 25×) duct dilation and (D) (H&E, 50×) distortion (arrows: inflammatory infiltrate) is characteristic of CP in histopathology. (Irene Esposito et., Guidelines on the histopathology of chronic pancreatitis. Recommendations from the working group for the international consensus guidelines for chronic pancreatitis in collaboration with the International Association of Pancreatology, the American Pancreatic Association, the Japan Pancreas Society, and the European Pancreatic Club, Pancreatology, 20(4), 2020, 586–593, https://doi.org/10.1016/j.pan.2020.04.009.)

Table 1
MRI/sMRCP findings for chronic pancreatitis

MRI Parenchymal Features	Secretin-Stimulated MRCP Features
Pancreatic atrophy (Mean anteroposterior diameter below the lower limit of age-related mean size)	Main pancreatic duct (MPD) irregularity
T1 signal-intensity ratio between pancreas and spleen	MPD dilation
T1 signal-intensity ratio between pancreas and paraspinal muscle	MPD stenosis
Presence of cysts	Presence of side branches
Duodenal filling-semiquantitative assessment of exocrine pancreatic function	
Grade 0—No fluid in the duodenum	
Grade 1—Fluid limited to the duodenal bulb	
Grade 2—Fluid filling up to genu-inferious	
Grade 3—Fluid filling beyond genu-inferious	

Abbreviations: CP, chronic pancreatitis; MRI, magnetic resonance imaging; sMRCP, secretin-stimulated MRCP.

Trikudanathan, Guru MD et al., FACG1 Diagnostic Performance of Contrast-Enhanced MRI With Secretin-Stimulated MRCP for Non-Calcific Chronic Pancreatitis: A Comparison With Histopathology, American Journal of Gastroenterology: November 2015 - Volume 110 - Issue 11 - p 1598–1606, https://doi.org/10.1038/ajg.2015.297.

resonance cholangiopancreatography (sMRCP) are used in conjunction with clinical presentation of chronic "pancreatic-type" abdominal pain to establish the diagnosis of noncalcific CP.[24,25]

Pancreatic tissue from patients with midstage CP as seen in TPIAT specimens have contributed to advancements in our understanding of the relationship between image-based criteria for CP and severity of fibrosis in noncalcified CP. Trikudanathan and colleagues[24,26] retrospectively evaluated 68 patients who underwent TPIAT for noncalcified CP. In their study, 4 or more EUS standard features optimized sensitivity (61%) and specificity (75%) to predict noncalcified CP. There was a poor correlation ($r = 0.2$, $P < .05$) between EUS standard features and histopathology, and the utility of EUS seemed to lie in the ability to predict the presence versus absence of fibrosis (AUROC 0.68 and accuracy of 63.2%).[24] Trikudanathan and colleagues[25] further retrospectively evaluated MRCP studies of 57 patients who underwent TPIAT for noncalcified CP to assess the correlation of MRCP with surgical histopathology in noncalcified CP. In their study, 48 patients with refractory abdominal pain and abnormal histology (fibrosis score ≥ 2) underwent MRCP within 1 year before TPIAT. Using a nonstandardized scoring system of potential MRI findings (Table 1), they found that the presence of 2 or more MRI/sMRCP features optimized sensitivity (65%, 95% CI: 49.5%–77.8%) and specificity (89%, 95% CI: 51.7%–98.2%) to predict abnormal histology (fibrosis score > 2) and was the best cutoff for the diagnosis of severe fibrosis (fibrosis score > 6), with a sensitivity of 88% (95% CI: 61.6%–98.1%) and specificity of 78% (95% CI: 62.4%–89.4%). There was a strong correlation between the number of MRI/sMRCP features and the fibrosis score ($r = 0.6$, $P < .0001$).[25]

SUMMARY

In summary, pancreatic tissue collected from patients undergoing TPIAT has provided valuable insight into the differences in histopathology of CP among patients with PRSS1 and SPINK1 mutations, immunohistologic differences between genetic and idiopathic CP while suggesting the potential for new tools such as RNASeq to define pathways contributing to the pathogenesis of alcoholic or hereditary CP, and allowing opportunities to validate noninvasive tools such as EUS and MRCP for the diagnosis of noncalcified CP.

CLINICS CARE POINTS

- Histology and immunologic research suggest that herediatry and non-hereditary pancreatitis may exhibit different immune inflitrates and pathologic changes.

- Diagnosis of early (non calcific CP) can be challenging. MRCP may be more sensitive and specific than EUS to diagnosis non-calcific CP, but an EUS score of 4 or more is also reasonably accurate at detecting early fibrosis.

DISCLOSURE

Dr S.M.B. Finn has nothing to disclose. Dr M.D. Bellin was supported by R01-DK109124 and also discloses relationships with Insulet (DSMB member), Ariel Precision Medicine (advisory board), and Viaycte (research support).

REFERENCES

1. Abu-El-Haija M, Anazawa T, Beilman GJ, et al. The role of total pancreatectomy with islet autotransplantation in the treatment of chronic pancreatitis: a report from the International Consensus Guidelines in chronic pancreatitis. Pancreatology 2020;20(4): 762–71.

2. Whitcomb DC, Frulloni L, Garg P, et al. Chronic pancreatitis: an international draft consensus proposal for a new mechanistic definition. Pancreatology 2016;16(2):218–24.

3. Yadav D, Lowenfels AB. The epidemiology of pancreatitis and pancreatic cancer. Gastroenterology 2013;144(6):1252–61.

4. Bellin MD, Kerdsirichairat T, Beilman GJ, et al. Total pancreatectomy with islet autotransplantation improves quality of life in patients with refractory recurrent acute pancreatitis. Clin Gastroenterol Hepatol 2016;14(9):1317–23.

5. Ammann RW. Diagnosis and management of chronic pancreatitis: current knowledge. Swiss Med Weekly 2006;136(11–12):166–74.

6. Gardner TB, Adler DG, Forsmark CE, et al. ACG clinical guideline: chronic pancreatitis. Am Coll Gastroenterol 2020;115(3):322–39.

7. Cahen DL, Gouma DJ, Nio Y, et al. Endoscopic versus surgical drainage of the pancreatic duct in chronic pancreatitis. N Engl J Med 2007;356(7):676–84.

8. McEachron KR, Bellin MD. Total pancreatectomy and islet autotransplantion for chronic and recurrent acute pancreatitis. Curr Opin Gastroenterol 2018;34(5): 367–73.

9. Wilhelm JJ, Balamurugan AN, Bellin MD, et al. Progress in individualizing autologous islet isolation techniques for pediatric islet autotransplantation after total pancreatectomy in children for chronic pancreatitis. Am J Transplant 2021;21(2):776–86.

10. Bellin MD, Beilman GJ, Sutherland DF, et al. How durable is total pancreatectomy and intraportal islet cell transplantation for treatment of chronic pancreatitis? J Am Coll Surg 2019;228(4):329–39.

11. Sacco Casamassima MG, Goldstein SD, Yang J, et al. The impact of surgical strategies on outcomes for pediatric chronic pancreatitis. Pediatr Surg Int 2017;33(1):75–83.

12. Chinnakotla S, Radosevich DM, Dunn TB, et al. Long-term outcomes of total pancreatectomy and islet auto transplantation for hereditary/genetic pancreatitis. J Am Coll Surg 2014;218(4):530–43.

13. Garcea G, Pollard CA, Illouz S, et al. Patient satisfaction and cost-effectiveness following total pancreatectomy with islet cell transplantation for chronic pancreatitis. Pancreas 2013;42(2):322–8.

14. Sutherland DE, Radosevich DM, Bellin MD, et al. Total pancreatectomy and islet autotransplantation for chronic pancreatitis. J Am Coll Surg 2012;214(4): 409–24.

15. Morgan KA, Lancaster WP, Owczarski SM, et al. Patient Selection for Total Pancreatectomy with Islet Autotransplantation in the Surgical Management of Chronic Pancreatitis. J Am Coll Surg 2018;226(4):446–51.

16. Esposito I, Hruban RH, Verbeke C, et al. Guidelines on the histopathology of chronic pancreatitis. Recommendations from the working group for the international consensus guidelines for chronic pancreatitis in collaboration with the International Association of Pancreatology, the American Pancreatic Association, the Japan Pancreas Society, and the European Pancreatic Club. Pancreatology 2020;20(4):586–93.

17. Klöppel G. Chronic pancreatitis, pseudotumors and other tumor-like lesions. Mod Pathol 2007;20(Suppl 1):S113–31.

18. Apte MV, Haber PS, Applegate TL, et al. Periacinar stellate shaped cells in rat pancreas: identification, isolation, and culture. Gut 1998;43(1):128–33.

19. Blobner BM, Bellin MD, Beilman GJ, et al. Gene Expression Profiling of the Pancreas in Patients Undergoing Total Pancreatectomy With Islet Autotransplant Suggests Unique Features of Alcoholic, Idiopathic, and Hereditary Pancreatitis. Pancreas 2020;49(8):1037–43.

20. Lee B, Adamska JZ, Namkoong H, et al. Distinct immune characteristics distinguish hereditary and idiopathic chronic pancreatitis. J Clin Invest 2020; 130(5):2705–11.

21. Singhi AD, Pai RK, Kant JA, et al. The histopathology of PRSS1 hereditary pancreatitis. Am J Surg Pathol 2014;38(3):346–53.

22. Jones TE, Bellin MD, Yadav D, et al. The histopathology of SPINK1-associated chronic pancreatitis. Pancreatology 2020;20(8):1648–55.

23. Kim DH, Pickhardt PJ. Radiologic assessment of acute and chronic pancreatitis. Surg Clin North Am 2007;87(6):1341–58, viii.

24. Trikudanathan G, Vega-Peralta J, Malli A, et al. Diagnostic Performance of Endoscopic Ultrasound (EUS) for Non-Calcific Chronic Pancreatitis (NCCP) Based on Histopathology. Am J Gastroenterol 2016;111(4): 568–74.

25. Trikudanathan G, Walker SP, Munigala S, et al. Diagnostic Performance of Contrast-Enhanced MRI With Secretin-Stimulated MRCP for Non-Calcific Chronic Pancreatitis: A Comparison With Histopathology. Am J Gastroenterol 2015;110(11):1598–606.

26. Trikudanathan G, Munigala S, Barlass U, et al. Evaluation of Rosemont criteria for non-calcific chronic pancreatitis (NCCP) based on histopathology - A retrospective study. Pancreatology 2017;17(1):63–9.

The Histopathology of Neoadjuvant-Treated (NAT) Pancreatic Ductal Adenocarcinoma

Ahmed Bakhshwin, MD[a], Daniela S. Allende, MD, MBA[b],*

KEYWORDS

• Pancreatic ductal adenocarcinoma • Neoadjuvant • Histology • Tumor response • Survival

Key points

- Recent neoadjuvant therapy regimens allow successful downstaging of borderline resectable and locally advanced pancreatic ductal adenocarcinoma and improve survival.
- The lack of standardized approach has led to great variations in tumor sampling, and tumor size assessment resulting in noncomparable data among different studies.
- Many different tumor regression grading systems are being used in clinical practice, all with advantages and limitations.

ABSTRACT

Examination of pancreatic ductal adenocarcinoma after NAT with the intent of diagnosis and outcome prediction remains a challenging task. The lack of a uniform approach to macroscopically assess these cases along with variations in sampling adds to the complexity. Several TRG systems have been proposed to correlate with an overall survival. In clinical practice, most of these TRG schemes have shown low level of interobserver agreement arguing for a need of larger studies and more innovative ways to assess outcome in this population.

OVERVIEW

Pancreatic carcinoma accounts for 3.2% of all new cancer cases in the United States and has a 5-year relative survival rate of 10.8% according to the Surveillance, Epidemiology, and End Results (SEERS) database.[1] For the purpose of this discussion, the article will focus on the most common form of pancreatic carcinoma, pancreatic ductal adenocarcinoma (PDAC). Most patients present with unresectable or locally advanced disease, and only up to one-third of patients are surgical candidates. In recent years, the introduction of neoadjuvant therapy (NAT) including regimens with FOLFIRINOX or gemcitabine-based with and without concomitant radiation have been successful in downstaging pancreatic ductal carcinoma in patients that are initially classified as "borderline" or "locally advanced" allowing for R0 resections in up to 63% of borderline resectable cases.[2] Despite the encouraging results, PDAC continues to represent 7.9% of all cancer-related death and is expected to become the second leading cause of cancer related death by 2030.[3] Considering that American Joint Commission on Cancer (AJCC) eighth edition tumor staging (pT) is based on tumor size to predict outcome, and tumor size is clearly affected

[a] Robert J. Tomsich Pathology & Laboratory Medicine Institute, Cleveland Clinic, 9500 Euclid Avenue, L1-360-R11, Cleveland, OH 44195, USA; [b] Robert J. Tomsich Pathology & Laboratory Medicine Institute, Cleveland Clinic, 9500 Euclid Avenue, L25, Cleveland, OH 44195, USA
* Corresponding author.
E-mail address: allendd@ccf.org
Twitter: @Ahmed_Bakhshwin (A.B.); @Allende_DS (D.S.A.)

surgpath.theclinics.com

by NAT, many unanswered questions remain: 1. What is the range of changes that can be expected in pancreatic carcinomas post-NAT? 2. Which grossing technique performs better in this setting? 3. What is the best way to measure tumor size and stage this population, and is tumor size a reliable prognostic parameter in these patients? 4. Which TRG system best correlates with outcome?

HANDLING NEOADJUVANT-TREATED PANCREATECTOMY SPECIMENS

MACROSCOPIC FINDINGS

Pancreatectomy specimens can be challenging in the grossing room given their complex anatomy, and that most centers have relative low volumes. Additional factors adding to the lack of standardized approach are the multiple grossing protocols available (axial, bivalving, and so forth), differences in sampling (representative sections, totally submitting the tumor/tumor bed, or entirely processing the pancreas), and characteristics of the tumor (often poorly circumscribed, and hard to differentiate from the adjacent fibrosis).[4] As a consequence of NAT, areas of tumor are replaced by fibrosis blurring the tumor boundaries. In most cases, the nontumoral parenchyma also displays variable degrees of fibrosis. This often makes identifying residual viable tumor and measuring tumor size extremely difficult or impossible even among trained pathologists.[5] The literature has used the term "tumor bed" to acknowledge that in this setting, distinguishing residual carcinoma from fibrosis is not a straightforward task. That said, gross examination and proper sampling remain critical for accurate pathologic condition evaluation and assessment of tumor regression.[5,6]

COMMONLY USED GROSSING TECHNIQUES FOR HANDLING PANCREATICODUODENECTOMY SPECIMENS

The bivalving and the axial sectioning protocols are the most frequently used around the world. Both methods and general recommendations on grossing these specimens have been previously described in detail elsewhere.[7,8] The bivalving method is adopted by most institutions in the United States, whereas the axial slicing method is widely used in Europe and Asia and was more recently introduced in the United States. In 2018, the Neoadjuvant Therapy Working Group of the Pancreatobiliary Pathology Society was formed. The working group includes expert pancreatic pathologists from around the world and aims to standardize the approach to these specimens. To date, there are

no strong recommendations regarding which grossing protocol should be used, and the decision is left to the comfort level of the pathologist handling the specimen. Recent studies comparing both approaches showed that both methods performed similarly; these methods are better than nonstandardized sampling and both have strengths and weaknesses.[9,10] Currently, literature is lacking large-scale studies that compare these 2 approaches in the setting of NAT.

For reference, a summary of standard sections of pancreaticoduodenectomy specimens and distal pancreatectomy are summarized in **Boxes 1** and **2**, respectively.

Independently of the method of choice, a few considerations are applicable to NAT-PDAC specimens:

Tumor Sampling, Tumor Size, and AJCC eighth Edition ypT Staging

Submitting representative sections versus entirely submitting the tumor remains a controversial point with lack of uniform agreement among pathologists. That said, studies in the field have shown better survival in cases with complete response or minimal evidence of residual viable tumor.[11–13] These data would support systematic mapping and more thorough sampling of tumors, which at many large centers includes submitting the tumor in toto. Some authors have proposed to submit tumor of up to 3 cm and add representative sections after that for larger tumors.[14] Although the approach is not yet standardized, demonstrating complete tumor response may have prognostic value in this population and may require submitting the entire pancreatic tissue, bile duct, and ampullary tissue/adjacent duodenal wall to document no residual disease. Studies have demonstrated that if this is the approach, the complete response rate is approximately 2.5% versus 10% to 33% when less extensive sampling is performed.[15] It is important to mention that in some cases of not residual carcinoma in the pancreas, scattered adenocarcinoma glands can be seen when the adjacent duodenal wall is sampled. The 2019 Amsterdam International Consensus meeting emphasized the need of prospective studies to determine the extent of adequate sampling in this setting.[16]

In the setting of NAT, the gross estimation of tumor size in pancreatic resection specimens may not always correspond with microscopic evidence of residual ductal adenocarcinoma. There is no reliable technique to differentiate residual tumor from tumor bed fibrosis secondary to therapy (**Fig. 1**). A study done on 289 NAT-PDAC cases revealed that gross tumor size alone did

---

Box 1
Summary of standard sections of pancreaticoduodenectomy

Tumor/tumor bed:

- $\leq$ 3 cm: entirely submit.

- Greater than 3 cm: sample extensively, with 1 tumor block per 0.5–1 cm interval

- Representative sections of tumor in relation to: common bile duct, Ampulla of Vater, duodenal mucosa, any other organs/anatomic landmarks present

Proximal gastric/duodenal margin (1 representative section)

Distal small bowel margin (1 representative section)

Pancreatic neck margin (entirely)

Common bile duct margin (entirely)

Superior mesenteric artery/uncinate margin (entirely)

Vascular groove (at least one section closest to tumor)

Anterior and posterior free surfaces (at least one section from each, closest to tumor)

If superior mesenteric vein/portal vein is present:

- Patch: ink the tips and submit in separate cassette(s); serially section the rest and entirely submit in relation to underlying tumor

- Segment: submit the superior and inferior vein margins en face in separate cassette(s); serially section the rest and entirely submit in relation to underlying tumor

Uninvolved pancreas (at least one section)

All possible lymph nodes

---

not provide adequate stratification based on AJCC eighth edition staging.[17] The current College of American Pathologists (CAPs) pancreatic cancer protocol recommends that gross assessment of tumor size be validated by microscopic examination for PDAC.[18] It seems that in most cases, the tumors do not "shrink" concentrically after NAT and scattered foci of residual viable carcinoma are noted throughout the fibrous tumor bed in cases with incomplete response.[15] Adopted from the international working group recommendations on standardized pathologic

evaluation of post-NAT breast cancer, Chatterjee and colleagues[11] proposed that the tumor size should be measured grossly and validated microscopically ("largest linear dimension"; **Fig. 2**). Based on this approach, the authors analyzed 398 NAT-PDAC and stated that the AJCC eighth edition ypT stage correlated with lymph nodes metastasis, tumor response grade, disease-free survival (DFS), and overall survival (OS). Interestingly, the authors proposed that a tumor size cutoff of 1.0 cm may be more reliable in predicting

---

Box 2
Summary of standard sections of distal pancreaticoduodenectomy

Tumor/tumor bed:

- 3 cm or lesser: entirely submit.

- Greater than 3 cm: sample extensively, with 1 tumor block per 0.5–1 cm interval.

- Tumor to adjacent organs (eg, spleen, vessels, and so forth).

Pancreatic resection margin (entirely)

Anterior and posterior free surfaces (at least one section from each, closest to tumor)

Uninvolved pancreas

All possible lymph nodes

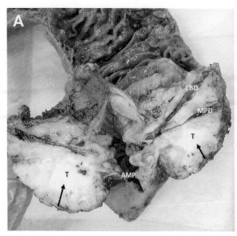
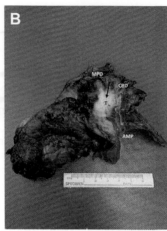

Fig. 1. (*A*) Macroscopic appearance of NAT-PDAC with ill-defined borders (*arrows*), difficult to distinguish tumor from the surrounding nonneoplastic tissue. (*B*) On the other hand, the tumor borders are easily discernible in the untreated (no NAT) setting. AMP, Ampulla of Vater; CBD, common bile duct; MPD, main pancreatic duct; T, tumor.

prognosis for ypT2 in comparison to the proposed tumor size cutoff of 2.0 cm.[19]

Lymph Node Dissection

The importance of appropriately and thoroughly examining the lymph nodes from pancreatectomy specimens cannot be overemphasized. Not only is it paramount for accurate determination of N staging but it also provides crucial prognostic information for patients with PDAC.[20–22] The minimum number of lymph nodes needed for accurate staging is at least 12 lymph nodes, according to CAP protocol and AJCC Cancer Staging Manual.[6] Considering the prognostic information obtained from lymph node metastasis, it seems reasonable to completely submit the peripancreatic fat and retroperitoneal soft tissue as described by the "orange peeling" methodology to maximize the lymph node detection rate.[23]

MICROSCOPIC FINDINGS

HISTOMORPHOLOGIC CHANGES ASSOCIATED WITH NEOADJUVANT-TREATED PANCREATIC CANCER

It is well accepted that NAT induces a wide range of morphologic changes. These changes have been well documented in a variety of organs, such as head and neck, stomach, and colorectal cancers.[24] However, this does not hold true for PDAC, where literature is sparse and mainly focuses on estimating the residual tumor volume. Nonetheless, it is imperative for practicing pathologists to be aware of these changes that are likely to be encountered to ensure proper identification of residual tumor and avoid pitfalls. A summary of most of these changes is listed in (Table 1).

Most available studies reported morphologic findings associated with either combination neoadjuvant chemoradiation or neoadjuvant chemotherapy alone. Only one study by Ishikawa and colleagues[25] reported findings with neoadjuvant radiotherapy alone. Hence, a head-to-head comparison between chemotherapy versus radiotherapy-related changes is difficult to discuss here.

Neoplastic Cells Changes

Overall, the morphologic changes induced by NAT in PDAC significantly overlap with those observed in other organs of the gastrointestinal tract. The nuclei of the neoplastic cells exhibit pyknosis (Fig. 3A), random nuclear atypia, and more pronounced hyperchromasia. These nuclear changes are usually accompanied by dense eosinophilic cytoplasm (Fig. 3B, C), which together represent the prototypical constellation seen with NAT. It is not uncommon to encounter other forms of cytoplasmic changes such as clear cell change, oncocytic change, rhabdoid change, vacuolization (Fig. 3D), and foamy cytoplasm (Fig. 3E).[26,27] In many instances, these features are seen intermixed in the same case or even the same gland. In clear cell change, the cells assume a pyramidal shape with ample clear cytoplasm and wrinkled, rasinoid nuclei. Vacuolization can range from a single, large vacuole pushing the nucleus to the periphery (signet ring-like), to multiple, smaller vacuoles encroaching on a centrally located nucleus (lipoblast-like). In contrast to eosinophilic change, the cells in oncocytic change have more abundant, granular cytoplasm, large, round, centrally located nuclei, and prominent nucleoli. Rhabdoid change occurs in a minority of cases and usually presents focally. The rhabdoid cells

Fig. 2. Proposed diagram of the tumor size measurement for neoadjuvant-treated pancreatic ductal adenocarcinoma. (*A*) With a single focus of viable residual tumor is present, the largest linear dimension of that focus should be used as the final tumor size. (*B*) When 2 or more foci are present, the largest linear dimension of the area involved by residual tumor, including the intervening stroma should be used. (*C*) When 2 or more foci are present and the residual tumor extends beyond the tumor bed area, the largest linear dimension of the entire area involved by residual tumor, including the intervening stroma, uninvolved pancreas, or peripancreatic soft tissue, should be used.

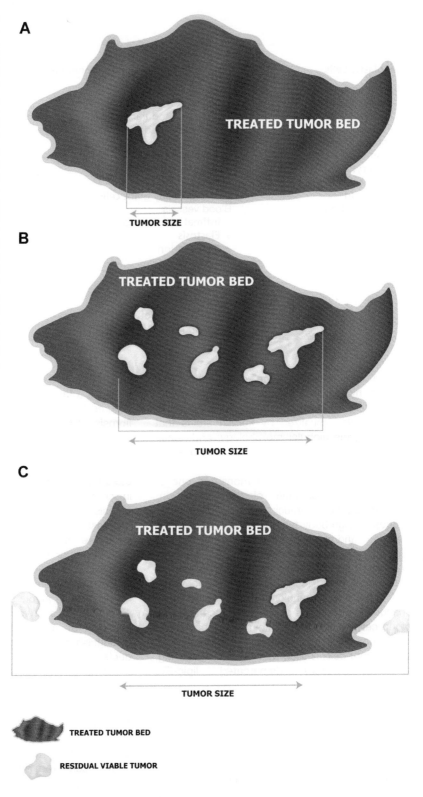

Table 1
Histologic changes following NAT in pancreatic ductal adenocarcinoma

Neoplastic Cells	Stroma/Inflammatory Environment	Nonneoplastic Tissue

Nuclear changes
• Hyperchromasia
• Bizarre nuclear atypia
• Pyknosis
Cytoplasmic changes
• Eosinophilic change
• Oncocytic change
• Clear cell change
• Rhabdoid
• Vacuolization
• Foamy cytoplasm
	Fibrosis
	• Loose fibromyxoid "blue/gray"
	• Cellular "nodular fasciitis-like"
	• Hypocellular, dense "keloid-like"
	Inflammation
	• Generally sparse
	• Lymphoplasmacytic
	• Foamy histiocytes ±
	  foreign body giant cells
	Blood vessels
	• Intimal hyperplasia
	• Elastosis
	• Obliteration
	Amyloid deposition
	Degenerative changes
	• Necrosis
	• Dystrophic calcifications
	• Cholesterol clefts
	• Mucin pool
		Lobular atrophy
		Islet cell aggregation
		Neural hyperplasia/"
		  neuroma-like" nerve
		  proliferations
		Squamous metaplasia

have a distinct appearance characterized by rounded, hyaline intracytoplasmic inclusions with eccentrically displaced nuclei. These inclusions can be better visualized by keratin stains that accentuate the globular morphology, and hence they are also referred to as "cytokeratin aggresome."[26]

Additionally, most cases demonstrate one or more of the following classic regression-associated features (mucin pool, foamy macrophages, foreign body-type giant cells, cholesterol clefts, and/or dystrophic calcification; **Fig. 4**A).[26,27] Finally, there are a few other changes that have been described in this setting, yet are rarely encountered, including erythrophagocytosis and "silicone granuloma-like" cytoplasmic change. The former is defined by discerning red blood cells or fragments within the cytoplasm of the tumor cells. In the latter, the cytoplasm of some tumor cells is filled with several coalescing, spherical, sharply demarcated lipid-like droplets.[26]

Stromal Fibrosis

In all studies that reported the histomorphologic findings of NAT PDAC, stromal fibrosis was a consistent observation. It is unclear whether the fibrosis is directly related to NAT, is part of tumor-induced desmoplasia, or is secondary to chronic pancreatitis. Regardless of the theory behind it, it is almost always present even in cases where NAT was not administered, which

supports some hypotheses that claim fibrosis provides a favorable microenvironment for tumor progression.[15,28,29] The interaction between the fibrosis and residual acinar parenchyma as well as residual tumor cells could serve as a diagnostic clue but also could be a potential pitfall. In the study by Vazzano and colleagues,[27] the authors reported that the blue/gray stromal fibrosis, in contrast to the classic dense eosinophilic fibrosis, was a helpful feature to locate residual neoplastic cells even at screening magnification. Extensive fibrosis can also overrun normal pancreatic parenchyma and distort benign ducts, mimicking a residual carcinoma. This can be further complicated when benign ducts show a mild degree of atypia secondary to the treatment effect. Careful examination of the architecture and cytology of glandular elements can typically distinguish tumor glands from atrophic, benign ducts.

Kalimuthu and colleagues reported 3 types of fibrosis based on the cellularity and the density of fibrosis as follows:

1. Paucicellular with loose and fibrotic to myxoid stroma (**Fig. 4**B).
2. Keloid-like"; hypocellular and dense fibrosis with scattered delicate fibroblasts (**Fig. 4**C). This type sometimes mimics the appearance of amyloid, which, can be separated by the absence of the characteristic amorphous quality of amyloid and the lack of staining with Congo red.

Fig. 3. Histologic changes in tumor cells after NAT. (*A*) Tumor cells displaying marked nuclear pyknosis and intracytoplasmic vacuole reminiscent of signet ring cells, (*B*) the neoplastic cells reveal marked cytoplasmic acidophilia and random nuclear atypia, and (*C*) neoplastic glands with dilated lumen and cytologic atypia including hyperchromasia and irregular nuclear membranes. Additional alterations commonly seen include:

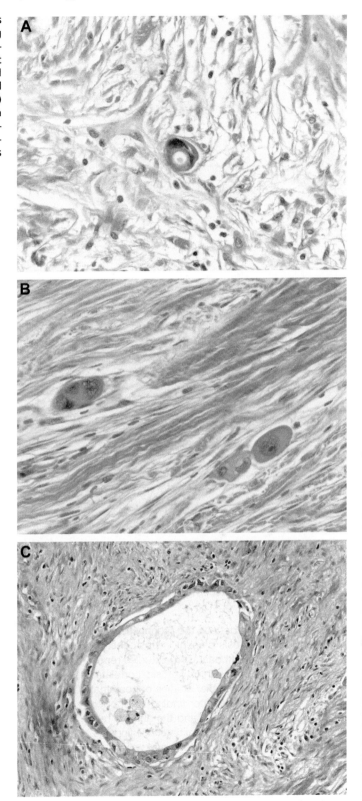

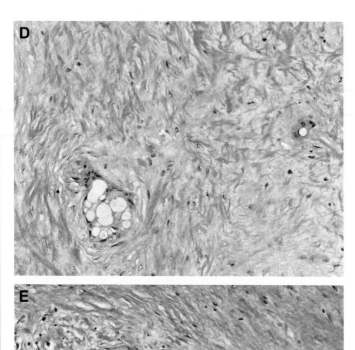

Fig. 3. (*continued*). (*D*) cytoplasmic vacuolization and (*E*) foamy cytoplasmic change.

3. 'Nodular fasciitis-like; moderately to markedly cellular stroma with accompanying granulation tissue formation (**Fig. 4**D).[26]

There is conflicting data on the prognostic value of the amount of fibrosis present in postpancreatectomy specimens. Although some studies report that an increased amount of fibrosis correlates with a better prognosis, other studies oppose that claim.[28,30] That said, the latter finding is reported in a small cohort of patients, and the authors recommended further studies to validate their findings. In a relatively recent study, Matuda and colleagues described a unique form of fibrosis, which they referred to as "encapsulating fibrosis" that is seen more frequently in patients who received NAT in contrast to patients who received adjuvant therapy after undergoing pancreatectomy. They defined encapsulating fibrosis as the formation of fibrous bands greater than 2 mm (diameter of the field,

using 10 × magnification) surrounding the neoplastic area. This histologic finding was associated with improved OS.[31]

There are additional changes that are not as common yet are unique to NAT-PDAC. Vazzano and colleagues found that vascular changes with intimal hyperplasia (**Fig. 4**E), obliterated lumen, and elastotic degeneration were seen in almost all NAT cohorts and none in the treatment-naïve group. Hemosiderin deposition can also be seen (**Fig.4**F). Similarly, islet amyloid deposition was an exclusive finding to the neoadjuvant-treated patients. Of note, the latter finding had no clear correlation with a history of diabetes mellitus.[27]

Inflammatory Environment

Inflammation following NAT varies and typically includes a combination of lymphocytes, foamy

Fig. 4. Stromal and vascular changes seen after NAT. (*A*) Giant cell reaction with cholesterol clefts. (*B*) scattered residual tumor cells embedded in a loose fibro-myxoid stroma, (*C*) neoplastic glands with treatment effect including attenuated epithelium and vacuolization, within dense hypocellular stroma with hyalinization and "keloid-like" fibers,

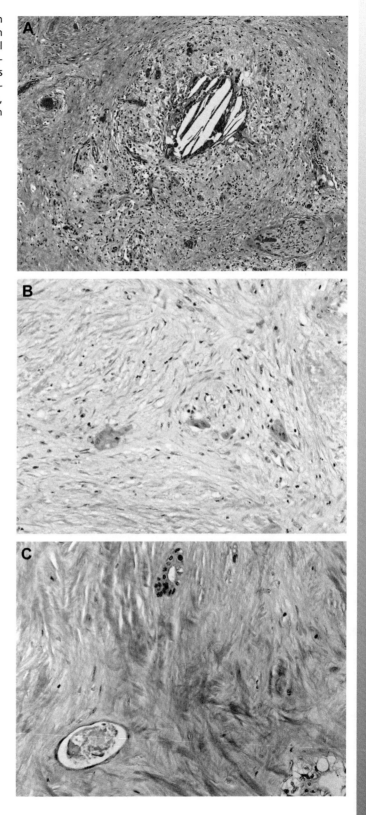

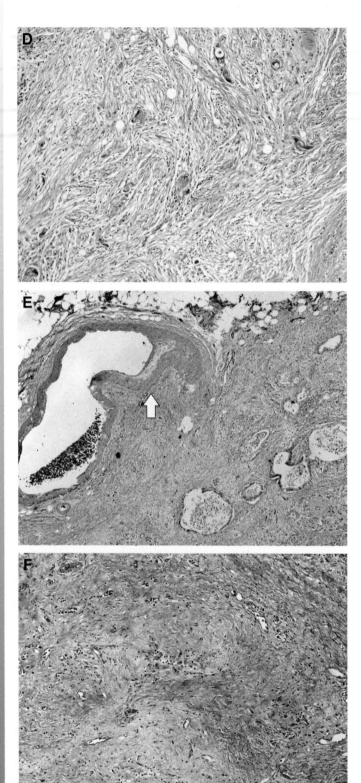

Fig. 4. (continued). (D) "nodular fasciitis-like" stromal changes, (E) focal intimal hyperplasia in an artery (arrow) adjacent to adenocarcinoma with treatment effect, and (F) scarring and hemosiderin deposition are common in areas of no residual tumor.

macrophages with scattered giant cells, plasma cells, and neutrophils, with lymphocytes being the most predominate inflammatory cell type. This inflammatory component can be subdivided into 2 locations: intratumoral (**Fig. 5**A) and peritumoral (within the nonneoplastic pancreas; **Fig. 5**B). In all studies to date, NAT seems to attenuate both types of the aforementioned inflammation. Data on the importance of intratumoral inflammation, particularly tumor infiltrating lymphocytes, after NAT is limited.[26,28,32] Nejati and colleagues[33] found that increased CD4+ lymphocytes are associated with reduced recurrence, longer DFS and OS, and is an independent prognostic factor for survival in patients with PDAC treated with NAT. Regarding the peritumoral inflammatory component, most studies have reported either no significant inflammation or only mild inflammation within the nonneoplastic pancreas. One group that found the presence of moderate-to-severe inflammation within the nonneoplastic parenchyma was associated with worse survival when compared with no or mild inflammation.[28] Recent studies demonstrated lower levels of FoxP3+ regulatory T cells and myeloid cells after NAT.[32,34] However, given the sparsity of literature on the topic of the significance of peritumoral and extratumoral inflammation, this remains an area requiring further investigation.

Alterations in the Nonneoplastic Pancreas

Neoadjuvant therapy also induces several changes within the nonneoplastic pancreas. Extensive fibrosis can result in significant lobular atrophy due to loss of exocrine pancreatic tissue (**Fig. 6**A). As a result, there is usually florid islet cell aggregation (**Fig. 6**B) that is particularly noticeable adjacent to the tumor. This can be quite striking and reach a size where one can contemplate the diagnosis of neuroendocrine microadenoma. Differentiating the 2 can be achieved by finding other islet cell aggregates of varying sizes in the vicinity, which are usually present with islet cell aggregation and not with microadenomas, and by demonstrating a polymorphous population of endocrine cells by retained expression of islet peptides on immunohistochemistry denoting a reactive proliferation and not a neoplasm. With significant background fibrosis and treatment changes, islet cells can assume a "single file" arrangement and closely aggregate next to nerves, simulating residual invasive cancer and perineural invasion (PNI).[26] In addition, neuroma-like nerve proliferation (**Fig. 6**C) characterized by disorganized and hypertrophied nerve bundles within fibrous stroma unrelated to PNI can also

be seen. Benign ducts may show squamous metaplasia. Finally, patients who received NAT seem to have less often high-grade pancreatic intraepithelial neoplasia (PanIN) in the background in comparison to those who did not receive NAT.[28]

GRADING TUMOR RESPONSE IN NAT-PANCREATIC DUCTAL ADENOCARCINOMA

Several TRG systems have been proposed for evaluating the extent of residual tumor in resections of PDAC following NAT. The 3 widely used grading systems are the Evans, CAP, and MD Anderson (MDA) systems (**Box 3**).[11,35,36] Each system has its methodological challenges and a certain degree of subjective interpretation of the categories described leading to low-level interobserver agreement. In most system, extensive sampling is required and residual tumor is often detected. Pathologists can select the TRG that they preferred. Regardless of the TRG system of choice, there is a uniform agreement among experts that regression grading is important to assess treatment response that is not captured by other histopathological parameters reported.[16] We will focus on covering these 3 main systems in detail and briefly outline more recently described grading systems.

EVANS GRADING SYSTEM

This system is the first of 2 TRG systems was originally published in 1992.[35] In their study, Evans and colleagues proposed estimating the overall destruction of neoplastic cells using a 4-tier system (grades I–IV). Necrosis is omitted for the grading scheme because it is often present in untreated tumors. This is the most extensively studied and used regression system in clinical trials. The major challenge when applying the Evans system is that it requires entire submission of the tumor bed for histologic review.

COLLEGE OF AMERICAN PATHOLOGISTS SYSTEM

The CAP TRG system is based on the modified Ryan scheme, which was originally proposed for treated rectal cancer.[36,37] Similar to the Evans system, it is a 4-tier grading scheme (0–3) based on estimating (eyeballing) the amount of residual viable tumor cells. This system is also used to evaluate tumor response for all other treated gastrointestinal carcinomas including esophagus, stomach, rectum, and anus. CAP protocol specifically indicates that other TRG systems can be

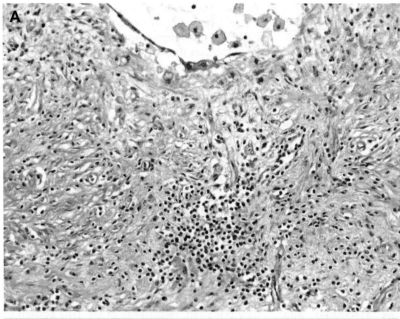

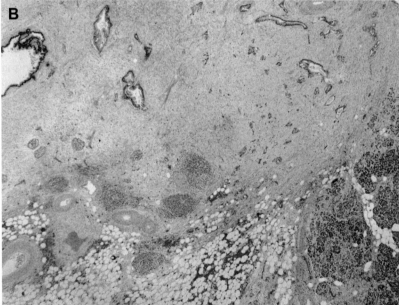

Fig. 5. Inflammatory environment in NAT-PDAC. (*A*) Intratumoral inflammatory response often includes lymphocytes, plasma cells, and histiocytes and (*B*) prominent lymphoid aggregates constitute peritumoral inflammatory response in some cases.

used. Nonetheless, it is imperative to clearly document which grading scheme was used in the CAP synoptic template, as well as in the pathology report. It is worth mentioning that the 2019 Amsterdam International Consensus Meeting endorsed the CAP system with the recommendation that the system should improve by using more objective parameters and replace some of the subjective terms such as "rare" and "extensive" that can lead to variability in interpretation among pathologists.[16]

Deshpande V and colleagues[38] compared the CAP TRG system to a quantitative assessment of tumor burden on whole slide scanned images and to semiquantitative analysis by eyeballing residual tumor in a cohort of 92 cases treated with FOLFIRINOX and radiation. A total of 16% achieved complete response, and 52% has less than 5% of residual tumor (in comparison to prior studies with gemcitabine that showed 2.5% of patients with complete response as pointed out by the authors). Interestingly, the authors noted that

Fig. 6. Histologic findings seen in the nonneoplastic parenchyma in NAT-PDAC cases. (*A*) Areas of exocrine parenchyma atrophy that remains in a lobular architecture with sparse ducts, neuroendocrine nests, and stromal fibrosis, (*B*) Islet cell aggregation as a result of pronounced atrophy of the pancreatic lobules, and (*C*) "neuroma-like" proliferation adjacent to arteries with intimal hyperplasia and luminal obliteration.

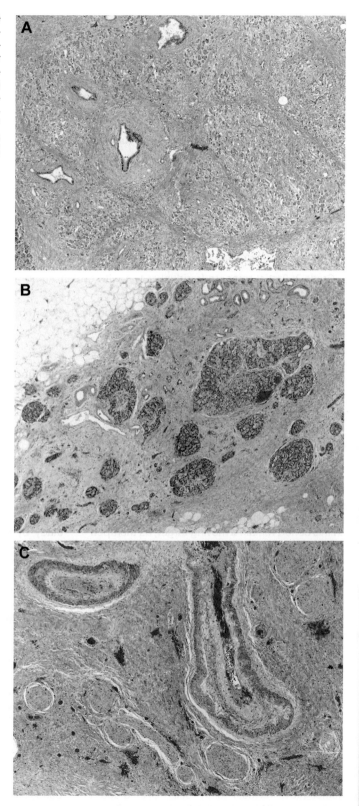

Box 3
Commonly used TRG schemes for NAT-pancreatic ductal adenocarcinoma

Evans Grading System (Percentage of tumor cell destruction)[35]

Grade I: Little (<10%) or no tumor cell destruction

Grade IIa: Destruction of 10%–50% of tumor cells

Grade IIb: Destruction of 51%–90% of tumor cells

Grade III: Few (<10%) viable-appearing tumor cells

- Grade IIIM: mucin pools with viable tumor cells

Grade IV: No viable tumor cells

- Grade IVM: Acellular pools of mucin

CAP Grading System (Amount of residual viable tumor cells)[36]

Grade 0: Complete response (no viable cancer cells)

Grade 1: Near complete response (single cells or rare small groups of cancer cells)

Grade 2: Partial response (residual cancer with evident tumor regression but more than single cells or rare small groups of cancer cells)

Grade 3: Poor or no response (extensive residual cancer with no evident tumor regression)

MDA Grading System (Percentage of viable tumor cells)[11]

Grade 0: No viable cancer cells (complete response)

Grade 1: Minimal residual carcinoma (single cells or small groups of cancer cells, <5% viable residual carcinoma)

Grade 2: 5% or more viable residual carcinoma cells

AJCC eighth edition was not predictive of outcome and improved survival in patients with up to 11.6% of residual tumor (as opposed to other studies suggesting a cut-off of 5%). These findings suggest that the parameters considered prognostic in this cohort remain a moving target, as therapeutic regimens continue to evolve. In this study, quantitative analysis on a single slide with the highest tumor burden (on multivariate and univariate analysis) correlated with OS, so did CAP TRG system (only on univariate analysis). The authors pointed out that using scanned slides for the assessment can be labor intensive and requires high-resolution scanners, so it may not be practical.

MD ANDERSON TRG SYSTEM

Chatterjee and colleagues[11] presented a 3-tier scheme that is modified from the Evans and the CAP systems, using 5% residual tumor cells as the critical cutoff. This cutoff was chosen after their study showed that patients with minimal residual tumor (<5% residual tumor cells, CAP grade 1, Evans grade III) had better DFS and OS. The authors reported similar findings in comparison to CAP TRG but easier applicability due to the 3-tiers.

Lee and colleagues[39] validated this TRG scheme on a large cohort of 167 PDAC patients who received NAT and subsequent pancreatoduodenectomy and reported improved interobserver agreement. This was also supported by a recent study by Kalimuthu and colleagues[40] who found that the MDA TRG system had the highest level of consensus among pathologists when compared with CAP or Evans TRG systems attributed by the authors to the "oversimplified" stratification. A downside of this system is that it classifies the majority (>80%) of PDAC patients as grade 2 response, which led the 2019 Amsterdam International Consensus to propose the CAP TRG scheme over the MDA system.[16]

Chetty and colleagues compared all 3 TRGs (Evans, CAP, and MDA) in a cohort treated with various chemotherapy regimens plus radiation and concluded that they lack precision and their clinical impact remains questionable.[40] A similar study by Kim and colleagues compared the same TRGs in cohort of 32 PDAC treated with neoadjuvant chemotherapy only (FOLFIRINOX and gemcitabine-based). The authors mentioned that in this setting, all 3 schemes were able to stratify patients in terms of overall and DFS.[41] Larger studies with standardized protocols may be needed to reach consensus.

Box 4
Less commonly used and some recently described TRG schemes

Ishikawa and colleagues (% of severely degenerated cancer cells [SDCCs] to cancer cells)[25]

Grade I: One-third or less SDCCs

Grade II: One-third to two-thirds SDCCs

Grade III: More than two-thirds SDCCs

White and colleagues (% viable tumor cells)[42]

Large: More than 90% viable tumor cells

Moderate: 10%–90% viable tumor cells

Small: less than 10% residual tumor cells

Minimal: Scattered foci of tumor cells

None: No residual tumor cells

Residual Tumor Index (% residual tumor x cm tumor bed size)[43]

Low: less than 0.2

Mid: 0.2–2

High: more than 2

Matsuda and colleagues; Area of Residual Tumor (viable tumor spanning 4× power objective fields)[44]

Score 0: No remaining viable cancer cells

Score 1: Viable tumor cells spanning ≤1 field, using 4× objective lens field

Score 2: Viable tumor cells spanning greater than 1 and ≤ 2 fields, using 4× objective lens field

Score 3: Viable tumor cells spanning greater than 2 and ≤ 3 fields, using 4× objective lens field

Score 4: Viable tumor cells spanning greater than 3 fields, using 4× objective lens field

Chou and colleagues; Royal North Shore (based on the % of tumor bed area occupied by viable carcinoma)[45]

Grade 1: 0%–10%

Grade 2: 11%–75%

Grade 3: 76%–100%

Other less commonly used and some newly proposed TRG systems are included in **Box 4.**[25,42–45]

Proposed prognostic factors (other than AJCC eighth edition ypT and TRG schemes) in NAT-PDAC.

- *Tumor invasion of muscular vessels is associated with poor prognosis:* Chatterjee and colleagues studied a cohort of 212 cases after NAT, 131 of them had lymphovascular space invasion and 30% of those showed invasion into muscular vessels. The latter was associated with positive margins, lymph node metastasis, locoregional/distant recurrence, and shorter overall and DFS.[46]
- *PNI and intraneural invasion carry poor prognosis:* In a series of 212 cases, PNI was identified in 58% of the 123 cases treated with

NAT. PNI was associated with tumor size, positive margins, lymph node involvement, and AJCC tumor stage. In particular, PNI or intraneural invasion correlated with shorter DFS and OS. On multivariate analysis, PNI was an independent predictor of outcome.[47]
- *A positive superior mesenteric artery (SMA) margin (SMAM) is associated with poor outcome:* In a series of 411 NAT-PDAC, 7.8% had positive margins based on CAP criteria. Margin-negative cases were further stratified as SMAM was 1 and lesser, 1.0 to 5.0, and greater than 5.0 mm. There was no difference in DFS or OS between the positive-margin group and SMAM≤1 mm. On multivariate analysis, SMAM distance, tumor grade, lymph node metastasis, and tumor

response grade were independent prognostic factors of DFS and OS. SMAM distance correlated with lower ypT and AJCC stage, greater tumor response, lower number of lymph node metastases, and less recurrence.[48]

- *Greater total number of lymph nodes involved is associated with poor prognosis*: Estrella and colleagues had shown that NAT-PDAC cases with 1 to 3 positive lymph nodes have better OS than patients with a greater number of positive lymph nodes.[13]
- *Tumor-insular complex are associated with poor treatment response in NAT-PDAC:* A recent study proposed the term tumor insular complex to characterize the intimate association between neoplastic ductal cells and non-neoplastic islet cells, which are reminiscent of ductulo-insular complexes.[49] The authors reviewed 105 cases and noted TIC in 33.3%. TIC was significantly associated with PNI, larger tumor bed size, percentage of residual tumor, residual tumor index, ypT stage, and poor treatment response.

SUMMARY

Examination of PDAC after NAT with the intent of diagnosis and outcome prediction remains a challenging task. The lack of a uniform approach to macroscopically assess these cases along with variations in sampling adds to the complexity. Several TRG systems have been proposed to correlate with OS. In clinical practice, most of these TRG schemes have shown low level of interobserver agreement arguing for a need of larger studies and more innovative ways to assess outcome in this population.

DISCLAIMER

Dr A. Bakhshwin has nothing to disclose. Dr D.S. Allende has participated as Advisory Board member for Incyte.

REFERENCES

1. Surveillance, epidemiology, and end results (SEER) program populations. National Cancer Institute, DCCPS, Surveillance Research Program; 2021. Available at: https://seer.cancer.gov/statfacts/html/pancreas.html. Accessed July 15, 2021.
2. Petrelli F, Coinu A, Borgonovo K, et al. FOLFIRINOX-based neoadjuvant therapy in borderline resectable or unresectable pancreatic cancer. Pancreas 2015; 44(4):515–21.
3. Rahib L, Smith BD, Aizenberg R, et al. Projecting cancer incidence and deaths to 2030: the unexpected burden of thyroid, liver, and pancreas cancers in the United States. Cancer Res 2014; 74(11):533–43.
4. Soer E, Brosens L, van de Vijver M, et al. Dilemmas for the pathologist in the oncologic assessment of pancreatoduodenectomy specimens. Virchows Arch 2018;472(4):483–90.
5. Nagaria TS, Wang H, Chatterjee D, et al. Pathology of treated pancreatic ductal adenocarcinoma and its clinical implications. Arch Pathol Lab Med 2020; 144(7):838–45.
6. Nagaria TS, Wang H. Modification of the 8th AJCC staging system of pancreatic ductal adenocarcinoma. Hepatobiliary Surg Nutr 2020;9(1):95–7.
7. Verbeke CS, Gladhaug IP. Dissection of pancreatic resection specimens. Surg Pathol Clin 2016;9(4): 523–38.
8. Adsay NV, Basturk O, Saka B, et al. Whipple made simple for surgical pathologists. Am J Surg Pathol 2014;38(4):480–93.
9. Grillo F, Ferro J, Vanoli A, et al. Comparison of pathology sampling protocols for pancreatoduodenectomy specimens. Virchows Arch 2020;476(5): 735–44.
10. van Roessel S, Soer EC, van Dieren S, et al. Axial slicing versus bivalving in the pathological examination of pancreatoduodenectomy specimens (APOLLO): a multicentre randomized controlled trial. HPB 2021;S1365-182X(21):00006-X.
11. Chatterjee D, Katz MH, Rashid A, et al. Histologic grading of the extent of residual carcinoma following neoadjuvant chemoradiation in pancreatic ductal adenocarcinoma. Cancer 2012;118(12):3182–90.
12. Zhao Q, Rashid A, Gong Y, et al. Pathologic complete response to neoadjuvant therapy in patients with pancreatic ductal adenocarcinoma is associated with a better prognosis. Ann Diagn Pathol 2012;16(1):29–37.
13. Estrella JS, Rashid A, Fleming JB, et al. Post-therapy pathologic stage and survival in patients with pancreatic ductal adenocarcinoma treated with neoadjuvant chemoradiation. Cancer 2012;118(1): 268–77.
14. Hartman DJ, Krasinskas AM. Assessing treatment effect in pancreatic cancer. Arch Pathol Lab Med 2012;136(1):100–9.
15. Verbeke C, Häberle L, Lenggenhager D, et al. Pathology assessment of pancreatic cancer following neoadjuvant treatment: Time to move on. Pancreatology 2018;18(5):467–76.
16. Janssen Bv, Tutucu F, van Roessel S, et al. Amsterdam International Consensus Meeting: tumor response scoring in the pathology assessment of resected pancreatic cancer after neoadjuvant therapy. Mod Pathol 2021;34(1):4–12.
17. Rowan DJ, Hartley CP, Aldakkak M, et al. Gross tumor size using the AJCC 8th ed. T staging criteria

does not provide prognostic stratification for neoadjuvant treated pancreatic ductal adenocarcinoma. Ann Diagn Pathol 2020;46:151485.

18. Burgart L, Chopp W, Dhanpat J. Protocol for the examination of specimens from patients with carcinoma of the pancreas 2021. Available at: https://www.cap.org/protocols-and-guidelines/cancer-reporting-tools/cancer-protocol-templates. Accessed July 19, 2021.

19. Chatterjee D, Katz MH, Foo WC, et al. Prognostic significance of new AJCC tumor stage in patients with pancreatic ductal adenocarcinoma treated with neoadjuvant therapy. Am J Surg Pathol 2017; 41(8):1097–104.

20. Fischer LK, Katz MH, Lee SM, et al. The number and ratio of positive lymph nodes affect pancreatic cancer patient survival after neoadjuvant therapy and pancreaticoduodenectomy. Histopathology 2016; 68(2):210–20.

21. House MG, Gönen M, Jarnagin WR, et al. Prognostic significance of pathologic nodal status in patients with resected pancreatic cancer. J Gastrointest Surg 2007;11(11):1549–55.

22. Showalter TN, Winter KA, Berger AC, et al. The influence of total nodes examined, number of positive nodes, and lymph node ratio on survival after surgical resection and adjuvant chemoradiation for pancreatic cancer: a secondary analysis of RTOG 9704. Int J Radiat Oncol Biol Phys 2011;81(5): 1328–35.

23. Adsay NV, Basturk O, Altinel D, et al. The number of lymph nodes identified in a simple pancreatoduodenectomy specimen: comparison of conventional vs orange-peeling approach in pathologic assessment. Mod Pathol 2009;22(1):107–12.

24. Sethi D, Sen R, Sen J, et al. Histopathologic changes following neoadjuvant chemotherapy in various malignancies. Int J Appl Basic Med Res 2012;2(2):111–6.

25. Ishikawa O, Ohhigashi H, Teshima T, et al. Clinical and histopathological appraisal of preoperative irradiation for adenocarcinoma of the pancreatoduodenal region. J Surg Oncol 1989;40(3):143–51.

26. Kalimuthu SN, Serra S, Dhani N, et al. The spectrum of histopathological changes encountered in pancreatectomy specimens after neoadjuvant chemoradiation, including subtle and less-well-recognised changes. J Clin Pathol 2016;69(6): 463–71.

27. Vazzano J, Frankel WL, Wolfe AR, et al. Morphologic changes associated with neoadjuvant-treated pancreatic ductal adenocarcinoma and comparison of two tumor regression grading systems. Hum Pathol 2021;109:1–11.

28. Chatterjee D, Katz MH, Rashid A, et al. Pancreatic intraepithelial neoplasia and histological changes in non-neoplastic pancreas associated with

neoadjuvant therapy in patients with pancreatic ductal adenocarcinoma. Histopathology 2013; 63(6):841–51.

29. Ueno H, Shinto E, Shimazaki H, et al. Histologic categorization of desmoplastic reaction: its relevance to the colorectal cancer microenvironment and prognosis. Ann Surg Oncol 2015;22(5): 1504–12.

30. Chun YS, Cooper HS, Cohen SJ, et al. Significance of Pathologic Response to Preoperative Therapy in Pancreatic Cancer. Ann Surg Oncol 2011;18(13): 3601–7.

31. Matsuda Y, Inoue Y, Hiratsuka M, et al. Encapsulating fibrosis following neoadjuvant chemotherapy is correlated with outcomes in patients with pancreatic cancer. PLoS One 2019;14(9): e0222155.

32. Shibuya KC, Goel VK, Xiong W, et al. Pancreatic ductal adenocarcinoma contains an effector and regulatory immune cell infiltrate that is altered by multimodal neoadjuvant treatment. PLoS One 2014;9(5):e96565.

33. Nejati R, Goldstein JB, Halperin DM, et al. Prognostic Significance of tumor-infiltrating lymphocytes in patients with pancreatic ductal adenocarcinoma treated with neoadjuvant chemotherapy. Pancreas 2017;46(9):1180–7.

34. Tsuchikawa T, Hirano S, Tanaka E, et al. Novel aspects of preoperative chemoradiation therapy improving anti-tumor immunity in pancreatic cancer. Cancer Sci 2013;104(5):531–5.

35. Evans DB. Preoperative chemoradiation and pancreaticoduodenectomy for adenocarcinoma of the pancreas. Arch Surg 1992;127(11):1335–9.

36. Kakar S, Shi C, Adsay NV, et al. Protocol for the examination of specimens from patients with carcinoma of the pancreas 2021. Available at: https://documents.cap.org/protocols/cp-gihepatobiliary--pancreas-exocrine-17protocol-4001.pdf. Accessed July 23, 2021.

37. Ryan R, Gibbons D, Hyland JMP, et al. Pathological response following long-course neoadjuvant chemoradiotherapy for locally advanced rectal cancer His-topathology 2005;47(2):141–6.

38. Neyaz A, Tabb ES, Shih A, et al. Pancreatic ductal adenocarcinoma: tumour regression grading following neoadjuvant FOLFIRINOX and radiation. Histopathology 2020;77(1):35–45.

39. Lee SM, Katz MHG, Liu L, et al. Validation of a proposed tumor regression grading scheme for pancreatic ductal adenocarcinoma after neoadjuvant therapy as a prognostic indicator for survival. Am J Surg Pathol 2016;40(12):1653–60.

40. N Kalimuthu S, Serra S, Dhani N, et al. Regression grading in neoadjuvant treated pancreatic cancer: an interobserver study. J Clin Pathol 2017;70(3): 237–43.

41. Kim SS, Ko AH, Nakakura EK, et al. Comparison of tumor regression grading of residual pancreatic ductal adenocarcinoma following neoadjuvant chemotherapy without radiation. Am J Surg Pathol 2019;43(3):334–40.

42. White RR, Xie HB, Gottfried MR, et al. Significance of histological response to preoperative chemoradiotherapy for pancreatic cancer. Ann Surg Oncol 2005;12(3):214–21.

43. Panni RZ, Gonzalez I, Hartley CP, et al. Residual tumor index. Am J Surg Pathol 2018;42(11):1480–7.

44. Matsuda Y, Ohkubo S, Nakano-Narusawa Y, et al. Objective assessment of tumor regression in post-neoadjuvant therapy resections for pancreatic ductal adenocarcinoma: comparison of multiple tumor regression grading systems. Scientific Rep 2020;10(1):18278.

45. Chou A, Ahadi M, Arena J, et al. A critical assessment of postneoadjuvant therapy pancreatic cancer regression grading schemes with a proposal for a novel approach. Am J Surg Pathol 2021;45(3):394–404.

46. Chatterjee D, Rashid A, Wang H, et al. Tumor invasion of muscular vessels predicts poor prognosis in patients with pancreatic ductal adenocarcinoma who have received neoadjuvant therapy and pancreaticoduodenectomy. Am J Surg Pathol 2012; 36(4):552–9.

47. Chatterjee D, Katz MH, Rashid A, et al. Perineural and intraneural invasion in posttherapy pancreaticoduodenectomy specimens predicts poor prognosis in patients with pancreatic ductal adenocarcinoma. Am J Surg Pathol 2012;36(3):409–17.

48. Liu L, Katz MH, Lee SM, et al. Superior mesenteric artery margin of posttherapy pancreaticoduodenectomy and prognosis in patients with pancreatic ductal adenocarcinoma. Am J Surg Pathol 2015; 39(10):1395–403.

49. González IA, Kang L-I, Williams GA, et al. Tumor-insular complex in neoadjuvant treated pancreatic ductal adenocarcinoma is associated with higher residual tumor. Am J Surg Pathol 2020;44(6): 817–25.

The Molecular Pathogenesis and Targeted Therapies for Cholangiocarcinoma

Nesteene Joy Param[a], Emily R. Bramel[b], Daniela Sia, PhD[b],*

KEYWORDS

- Cholangiocarcinoma • Targeted therapies • Molecular aberrations • Microenvironment
- Precision medicine

Key points

- The incidence of cholangiocarcinoma (CCA) is on the rise.
- Despite some progress in our understanding of the molecular pathogenesis and treatment, patients' prognosis for CCA remains dismal.
- The identification of recurrent molecular alterations (ie, IDH mutations and FGFR2 fusions) has led to the Food and Drug Administration (FDA)-approval of the first-targeted therapies.
- Deeper understanding of the intricate relationship between the tumor cells and the surrounding microenvironment is becoming critical for the development of more effective therapeutic approaches.

ABSTRACT

Cholangiocarcinoma (CCA) is a group of malignancies of the bile ducts with high mortality rates and limited treatment options. In the past decades, remarkable efforts have been dedicated toward elucidating the specific molecular signaling pathways and oncogenic loops driving cholangiocarcinogenesis to ultimately develop more effective therapies. Despite some recent advances, an extensive intra- and inter-tumor heterogeneity together with a poorly understood immunosuppressive microenvironment significantly compromises the efficacy of available treatments. Here, we provide a concise review of the latest advances and current knowledge of the molecular pathogenesis of CCA focusing on clinically relevant aberrations as well as future research avenues.

INTRODUCTION

Owing to its aggressiveness and refractory nature, cholangiocarcinoma (CCA) is an intractable malignancy of the biliary tract with dramatically increasing incidence rates and dismal prognosis. Based on the anatomic position of origin, CCAs can be classified as intrahepatic CCA (iCCA) and extrahepatic CCA (eCCA), with iCCA arising from the bile ductules and second-order bile ducts within the liver and eCCA from the common bile duct.[1] In addition, eCCA can be divided into two distinct subtypes: perihilar, originating from the

[a] Department of Oncological Sciences, Tisch Cancer Institute, Icahn School of Medicine at Mount Sinai, 1425 Madison Avenue, 11th Floor Room 70-E, New York, NY 10029, USA; [b] Division of Liver Diseases, Department of Medicine, Tisch Cancer Institute, Icahn School of Medicine at Mount Sinai, 1425 Madison Avenue, 11th Floor Room 70-E, New York, NY 10029, USA
* Corresponding author.
E-mail address: daniela.sia@mssm.edu

Surgical Pathology 15 (2022) 529–539
https://doi.org/10.1016/j.path.2022.05.006

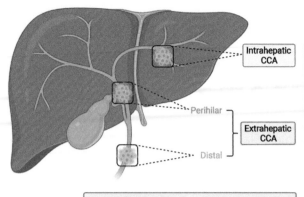

Fig. 1. Anatomic and molecular differences between iCCA and eCCA. CCAs include intrahepatic and extrahepatic CCA. Extrahepatic tumors can be subclassified into perihilar and distal tumors. Molecular alterations differ across the distinct subtypes. Here, we indicate some of the most common alterations as per previous report in *Valle and colleagues 2017*[66]. (*Courtesy of Biorender.*)

perihilar bile ducts and distal, originating from the common bile duct[1] (Fig. 1). Together, perihilar and distal CCA (herein eCCA) make up ~80% of all CCAs while iCCA account for 20%. Apart from the anatomic location, the differences between iCCA and eCCA extend to risk factors, cell(s) of origin, molecular aberrations, and clinical management.[1,2] Of note, incidence and mortality rates of CCA, particularly iCCA, have been steadily rising over the past 40 years,[3] highlighting the severity of the problem.

Despite increased understanding of the molecular pathogenesis has led to the identification of novel targets amenable to therapeutic intervention, the outlook for CCA remains grim.[4] CCAs tend to be asymptomatic in their early stages and most patients (~70%) are diagnosed when the disease has already metastasized.[1,4] Late diagnosis compromises the efficacy of surgical resection which currently represents the only curative option for patients with CCA.[4] For patients with unresectable tumors, palliative chemotherapy with gemcitabine plus cisplatin is the first-line treatment with a median overall survival of roughly 12 months.[1] Recently, isocitrate dehydrogenase (IDH) and fibroblast growth factor receptor 2 (FGFR2) inhibitors have shown some success in CCA, although the survival benefit conferred by these therapies remains modest. These data underscore the critical need for a deeper understanding of the molecular pathogenesis of CCA to identify treatment options that may help improving patients' prognosis. In this review, we detail the signaling pathways, genetic, and epigenetic aberrations leading the tumorigenesis and progression of CCA, whenever possible, we highlight molecular differences between iCCA and eCCA with particular emphasis on their clinical implications.

MOLECULAR PATHOGENESIS OF CHOLANGIOCARCINOMA

There is general consensus that CCAs can originate from the neoplastic transformation of cholangiocytes, hepatocytes, and/or progenitor cells.[2,5] An inflamed and highly desmoplastic microenvironment contributes to cholangiocarcinogenesis in a complex multistep process involving the activation or inactivation of specific pathways in the cell(s) of origin.[1,2] Although the process is still far from being fully understood, the identified cellular and non-cellular elements have long being recognized as valid targets for potential therapeutic opportunities.

SIGNALING PATHWAYS

INTERLEUKIN-6/ SIGNAL TRANSDUCER AND ACTIVATOR OF TRANSCRIPTION 3 (STAT3) SIGNALING

Chronic inflammation and fibrosis have been demonstrated to facilitate neoplastic transformation and growth mostly due to the secretion of several cytokines including interleukin-6 (IL6).[4] IL-6 expression is normally induced by tissue damage or stress, however, in CCA can be secreted by CCA cells in an autocrine and paracrine manner.[6] IL-6 provides a pro-tumoral effect on CCA tumor cells by inhibiting apoptosis and autophagy and inducing epithelial–mesenchymal transition (EMT). IL-6 upregulates AKT serine/threonine kinase (AKT) and myeloid leukemia 1 (MCL-1), which led to diminished TNF-related apoptosis-inducing ligand (TRAIL)-mediated apoptosis.[7] In CCA patients, high expression of IL-6 in the serum has been correlated with tumor burden and was found to be higher in patients with CCA compared with hepatocellular carcinoma (HCC).[8] *In vivo* and *in vitro* studies have shown that IL-6 blockade slows the progression of CCA.[9] Unfortunately, clinical trials using IL-6 blocking antibodies like siltuximab have shown no or only modest response to IL-6 therapy.

DEVELOPMENTAL PATHWAYS

The NOTCH signaling plays an essential role in the biliary tree development.[10] NOTCH aberrations have been implicated in several liver disorders, including hepatoblastoma (HB), HCC, and all subtypes of CCA.[11] Overall, 64% to 75% of NOTCH pathway genes have been found aberrantly expressed in CCA compared with the surrounding liver tissue.[12] In eCCA patients, the presence of at least one mutation of *NOTCH receptors 1-3* has been associated with poorer survival.[13] Overexpression of the activated form of *Notch receptor 1* (NOTCH1) in cooperation with AKT serine/threonine kinase 1 (AKT1) activation can mediate the trans-differentiation of hepatocytes into cholangiocytes and leads to iCCA formation in mice.[14]

The HIPPO signaling pathway is composed of kinase modules, macrophage stimulating 1 (MST1), macrophage stimulating 2 (MST2), large tumor suppressor kinase 1 (LATS1), and large tumor suppressor kinase 2 (LATS2), their regulator salvador family WW domain containing protein 1 (SAV1), and transcriptional modules, yes1 associated transcriptional regulator (YAP1) and tafazzin (TAZ). YAP1 and TAZ are transported between the nucleus and the cytoplasm where, through their interaction with the transcription factors, TEA domain transcription factor 1-4 (TEAD1-4), they induce cell proliferation and antiapoptotic genes.[15] In iCCA, YAP1 induces the transcription upregulation of *ankyrin repeat domain 1 (ANKRD1)*, *cellular communication network factor 1 (CYR61)*, and *connective tissue growth factor (CTGF)* which lead to increased tumor growth and downregulation of the proapoptotic TNF Superfamily Member 10 (TNFSF10)-TRAIL axis.[16] Upregulation of the histone methyltransferase G9a has also been shown to induce silencing of *LATS2* and aberrant YAP1 activation.[17] *YAP1* and *TAZ* expression in the tumor microenvironment (TME) can also affect the fate of the tumor. A study by Moya and colleagues[18] elegantly demonstrated that peritumoral hepatocytes express *YAP1* and *TAZ*, and deletion in these cells leads to accelerated growth and hyperactivation leads to regression.

WNT/β signaling is an essential component in the developmental process and is usually inactivated in normal adult tissue. Aberrant WNT/β signaling has been involved in the initiation and progression of HCC, CCA, and HB. Multiple WNT/β signaling components could be altered to cause tumor progression, including downregulation of secreted frizzled-related proteins, upregulation of WNT ligands, β-catenin scaffold proteins, and kinases.[19] Unlike HCC, mutations in the β-catenin (*CTNNB1*) gene have been rarely described in CCA.[20] Aberrant activity of other key proteins, such as nuclear receptor subfamily 4 group A member 2 (NR4A2) and osteopontin (OPN), has been shown to use WNT/β signaling to increase CCA tumor burden. OPN specifically reacts with β-catenin through the mitogen-activated protein kinase kinase MEK-MAPK1 pathway to mediate the phosphorylation and nuclear translocation of β-catenin to further increase downstream effector targets.[21] Another protein upstream of OPN, NR4A2, has been shown to upregulate OPN and WNT/β-catenin signaling, further reinforcing its pro-tumoral effect.[22]

Although these developmental pathways play an essential role in CCA progression, targeting them has been difficult. Considering that these pathways are essential for development and stem cell maintenance, their therapeutic inhibition may affect normal tissue regeneration.[23] In a clinical trial testing, a γ-Secretase inhibitor, 84% of patients experienced at least one treatment-related adverse event.[24] Modulating the toxicity of these therapies and understanding the crosstalk between the pathways will allow for more effective targeting of these networks.

RECEPTOR TYROSINE KINASE PATHWAYS

Deregulation of receptor tyrosine kinases (RTKs) is a shared feature among all CCA subtypes. Aberrant signaling via epidermal growth factor receptor (EGFR), vascular endothelial growth factor receptor (VEGFR), and fibroblast growth factor receptor 2 (FGFR2) leads to proliferation and survival through activation of the RAS-MAPK and PI3K-AKT. In addition, activating mutations of kirsten rat sarcoma viral oncogene homolog (*KRAS*), which occur in 25% to 30% across CCA subtypes, further increase RAS-MAPK signaling. Although aberrant RTK pathways represent valid actionable molecular targets, over the years results from phase I–II clinical studies testing TK inhibitors such as sorafenib, erlotinib, and cetuximab have been discouraging.

For example, a phase I study testing afatinib, a potential therapy that blocks downstream EGFR signaling, in combination with gemcitabine/cisplatin in patients with CCA was discontinued due to the lack of response and adverse events.[25] Interestingly, high levels of ROS proto-oncogene 1 (ROS1)/anaplastic lymphoma receptor tyrosine kinase (ALK)/hepatocyte growth factor receptor (c-MET), (RAM) in patients treated with gemcitabine plus oxaliplatin (GEMOX) with or without cetuximab, an EGFR inhibitor, have been found associated with shorter median overall survival compared with patients with low expression of RAM (5.7 vs 11.7 months),[26] suggesting RAM as a potential mechanism of resistance to EGFR therapies. These studies show the importance of identifying molecular markers of response and/or resistance for improved patient selection.

Tumor angiogenesis has been explored extensively in CCA. Unfortunately, targeted therapies aimed at attenuating angiogenesis, such as lenvatinib and cabozantinib, have been discouraging when administered to all comers. In a phase II clinical trial of lenvatinib, overall response rate (ORR) was confirmed only in 11.5% patients, with an overall survival of 7.35 months[27], whereas bevacizumab is currently in a phase III trial testing the drug in patients with inoperable biliary tract cancers.[28] In HCC, promising results have been seen in clinical trials studying lenvatinib in combination with PD-1 blockade.[29] Similar studies are being applied in clinical trials treating CCA (NCT04550624, NCT03951597, NCT03895970, and NCT05010668, **Fig. 2** and **Table 1**).

THE CHOLANGIOCARCINOMA MICROENVIRONMENT

The TME of CCA is made up of several distinct cell types including fibroblasts, immune cells, and extracellular matrix proteins (**Fig. 3**). Among the most studied are cancer-associated fibroblasts (CAFs). The abundance of CAFs in CCA patients has been associated with reduced overall survival.[30] CAFs promote CCA tumor growth by inducing a variety of cytokines and growth factors, including vascular endothelial growth factor (VEGF), fibroblast growth factor 2 (FGF2), and IL-6.[31] Recently, multiple subtypes of CAFs have been described by applying single-cell technologies in both human and murine CCA samples.[32,33] The dominant populations, myofibroblastic CAFs and inflammatory CAFs, are derived from hepatic stellate cells and interact with the tumor to promote tumor progression in iCCA.[32] Vascular CAFs have high expression of IL-6 and induce epigenetic alterations in iCCA tumor cells, while antigen-presenting CAFs have been shown to present antigens to CD4+ T cells to regulate the immune response.[33]

CCA tumors also have a diverse variety of immune cells.[31,33] Patients with high numbers of tumor-associated macrophages and regulatory T cells (Tregs) show a higher recurrence and low overall survival rates.[34,35] Despite positivity for programmed cell death ligand 1 (PD-L1) has been reported in about 10% to 60% of iCCA and eCCA tumors,[36] early clinical trials testing immune checkpoint inhibitors (ICIs) targeting the PD1/PD-L1 axis in unselected CCA populations have been disappointing.[37]

MOLECULAR CLASSIFICATIONS

Over the years, the generation of integrative molecular classifications of CCA has significantly contributed to our understanding of the molecular pathogenesis of both iCCA and eCCA. Regarding iCCA, there is large consensus that according to the transcriptional profile of the tumor, it can be divided into two main prognostic classes[38,39] named *inflammation* and *proliferation* (**Fig. 4**). The *inflammation class* (40% of all patients) is characterized by immune-related signaling pathways, whereas the *proliferation class* represents the activation of multiple oncogenic addiction pathways (ie, RTKs, NOTCH, and so forth), enrichment of *V-Raf murine sarcoma viral oncogene homolog B1 (BRAF)/RAS* mutations, high level amplification at 11q13, and poor outcome. The *proliferation class* also encompasses a subtype of iCCA with stem cell features,[40] chromosomal instability, and isocitrate dehydrogenase *(NADP(+)) 1/2 (IDH1/2)* mutations.

eCCA remains significantly underexplored compared with iCCA and to date only one molecular classification has been proposed for this subtype. Based on the analysis of gene expression and structural genomic aberrations of 189 clinically annotated eCCAs (76% pCCA and 24% dCCA), four distinct eCCA molecular classes have been described (see **Fig. 4**), namely (1) *metabolic*; (2) *proliferation*; (3) *mesenchymal*; and (4) *immune*.[41] Tumors classified within the *metabolic class* (19%) are enriched with gene signatures defining bile acid metabolism, whereas the *proliferation class* (23%) is associated with papillary histology and enrichment of several oncogenic pathways including MYC, mTOR, and ERBB2 signaling. The *mesenchymal class* (47%) is characterized by EMT, stromal activation, and poor outcome. Finally, tumors classified as *immune class* (12%) overexpress programmed cell death

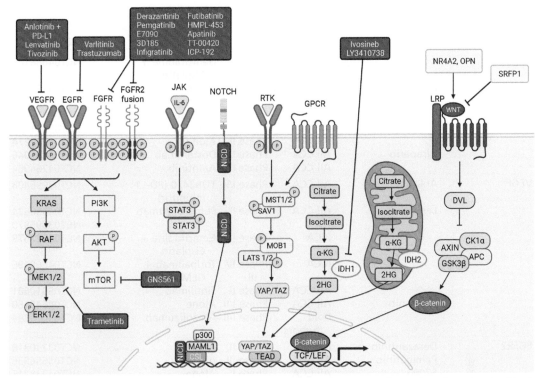

Fig. 2. *Molecular pathways and targeted therapies for CCA.* Several signaling pathways have been involved in the cholangiocarcinogenesis process and selective targeted therapies are currently being investigated in clinical trials (see Table 1). (*Adapted from* "The Tumor Microenvironment: Overview of Cancer-Associated Changes," *by* Bio-Render.com [2021]. *Retrieved from* https://app.biorender.com/biorender-templates.)

1 (PD1)/PD-L1 show higher presence of tumor-infiltrating lymphocytes and signatures predicting response to ICIs. Direct comparison of eCCA with previously described iCCA molecular classes identified significant similarities only in the two proliferation classes further delineating the differences between iCCA and eCCA. Albeit useful, molecular classifications of iCCA and eCCA have not yet been incorporated in clinical practice.

Considering the seminal role of the TME in dictating tumor behavior and response to therapies, the first genomic studies aimed at generating more comprehensive molecular classifications able to integrate elements of the tumor with immune and stroma features have started to emerge.[42,43] In this regard, we have recently described that iCCA can be divided into five distinct TME-based classes encompassing both inflamed and non-inflamed phenotypes. Overall, most of the iCCAs (>60%) resemble cold tumors with paucity of T cells and enrichment of immuno-suppressive elements, such as macrophages type 2 and Tregs, associated with specific structural aberrations.[43] On the other hand, the inflamed clusters account for less than 40% and differ in their signaling pathways, driver genes, and CAF

subtypes.[43] Validity of this novel stratification for the rationale design of combination of targeted therapies plus immunotherapies needs further validation in prospective clinical trials.

TARGETING THE MUTATIONAL LANDSCAPE OF CHOLANGIOCARCINOMA

The benefit of targeted therapies for patients with cancer, including CCA, is indisputable. A meta-analysis of seven randomized clinical trials showed higher ORR in patients with CCA treated with targeted therapy *plus* chemotherapy versus patients treated with chemotherapy alone.[44] However, the alignment between the molecular alteration and treatment efficacy is still imperfect. Overall, in CCA, 47% of all patients harbor actionable onco-genes and 39% present a mutation classified as level 3 using the precision oncology knowledge database OncoKB.[45] Potential targets include, phosphatidylinositol-4,5-bisphosphate 3-kinase catalytic subunit alpha (PIK3CA) and Erb-B2 receptor tyrosine kinase 2 (ERBB2).[45] With the exception of mutations in the *IDH1/2* gene and *FGFR2* fusions, most of these alterations occur only in a small

Table 1
Active clinical trials with targeted therapies in cholangiocarcinoma

Targets	Drug	CCA Type	Phase	Combination	Clinical Trial
IDH	Ivosidenib	All CCA	Phase I	Gemcitabine + Cisplatin	NCT04088188
	LY3410738	All CCA	Phase I	Alone	NCT04521686
	Olaparib	All CCA	Phase II	Pembrolizumab	NCT04306367
		All CCA	Phase II	Ceralasertib	NCT03878095
		All CCA	Phase II	Durvalumab	NCT03991832
		All CCA	Phase II	Alone	NCT03212274
	Niraparib	All CCA	Phase II	Dostarlimab	NCT04895046
		All CCA	Phase I	Anlotinib	NCT04764084
VEGF	Anlotinib	All CCA	Phase I/II	TQB2450 (PD-L1 inhibitor)	NCT03996408
	Lenvatinib	All CCA	Phase II	Pembrolizumab	NCT04550624 NCT03895970
		iCCA	Phase II	Gemcitabine + Cisplatin	NCT04527679
		iCCA	Phase II/III	Toripalimab + GEMOX	NCT04669496
		All CCA	Phase II	Sintilimab	NCT05010681
	Tivozanib	All CCA	Phase I/II	Alone	NCT04645160
		Cold tumors	Phase I/II	Atezolizumab	NCT05000294
FGFR2	Derazantinib	iCCA	Phase II	Alone	NCT03230318
	Pemigatinib	All CCA	Phase III	Alone	NCT03656536
	E7090	All CCA	Phase II	Alone	NCT04238715
	3D185	All CCA	Phase II	Alone	NCT05039892
	Infigratinib	All CCA	Phase II	Alone	NCT02150967
		All CCA	Phase III	Alone	NCT03773302
		All CCA	Phase II	Alone	NCT04233567
	Futibatinib	iCCA	Phase III	Alone	NCT04093362
	HMPL-453	iCCA	Phase II	Alone	NCT04353375
	Apatinib	iCCA	Phase II	Camrelizumab	NCT04454905
		iCCA	Phase II	DEB TACE + PD-1 Antibody	NCT04834674
	TT-00420	All CCA	Phase II	Alone	NCT04919642
	ICP-192	All CCA	Phase I/II	Alone	NCT04565275
	RLY-4008	All CCA	Phase I	Alone	NCT04526106
Sphingosine kinase	ABC294640	All CCA	Phase II	Hydroxychloroquine	NCT03377179
TGFB/COX	STP705	All CCA	Phase I	Alone	NCT04676633
TGFBRII	TGFBRII/PDL1 (M7824	All CCA	Phase II	Alone	NCT03833661
PPT1	GNS561	iCCA	Phase I/II	Alone	NCT03316222
ATR	Ceralasertib	All CCA	Phase II	Durvalumab	NCT04298008
MEK	Trametinib	All CCA	Phase II	Hydroxychloroquine	NCT04566133
TRAILR2	BI 905711	All CCA	Phase I	Alone	NCT04137289

Abbreviations: ATR, ataxia telangiectasia and Rad 3; TGFB, Transforming growth fcator beta.

fraction of CCA patients (<10%), favoring their enrollment in basket trials such as patients with TRK fusions.[46]

IDH1 AND *IDH2* MUTATIONS

IDH mutations occur in 15% to 20% of CCAs and are more commonly found in iCCA than eCCA.[47]

IDH mutations can alter cell differentiation, cell survival, and extracellular matrix maturation. Mechanistically, these mutations produce the ability to convert alpha ketoglutarate to 2-hydroxyglutarate (2HG). The 2HG production leads to the suppression of hepatocyte nuclear factor 4 alpha (HNF-4a), a transcription factor that regulates hepatocyte differentiation, which ultimately can lead

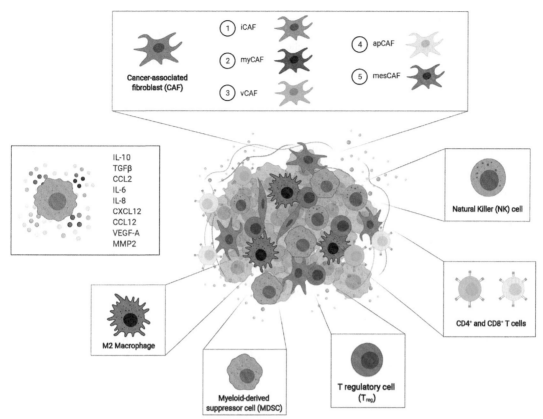

Fig. 3. *The tumor microenvironment of CCA.* CCA represents a complex tumor microenvironment comprising a mixture of cell types, including malignant cholangiocytes, immune cells, fibroblasts, and endothelial cells dispersed within the extracellular matrix and abundant supporting stroma. Although the immunobiology of iCCA remains poorly understood, the application of single-cell technologies and functional studies in murine models has contributed to elucidate the role of CAFs and identified distinct subtypes with specific functions. (*Adapted from* "Ras Pathway," by BioRender.com (2021). Retrieved from https://app.biorender.com/bio-render-templates.)

	Intrahepatic CCA		Extrahepatic CCA			
	Proliferation (60%)	Inflammation (40%)	Metabolic (19%)	Proliferation (23%)	Mesenchymal (47%)	Immune (11%)
Subtype	Progenitor-like		Hepatocyte-like phenotye			
Signalling Pathways	KRAS/RAF/ERK, IGF1R, EGFR, NOTCH, HER2, MET, PI3K/AKT/mTOR	Inflammatory pathways (Interleukins/chemokines), STAT3 activation	Metabolic pathways	mTOR, cell cycle, DNA repair	Hedgehog, TNFA, TGFB	Inflammatory pathways (IFN, PD1, etc)
Oncogenic Mutations	KRAS, BRAF, EGFR			ERBB2		
	IDH1/2					
	Chromatin remodelling genes (ARID1A, BAP1, PBMR1), TP53			KRAS/TP53/ARID1A/SMAD4		
Structural Aberrations	Chr 11q13 amplif. (CCND1, FGF19)					
	Chr14q22.1 (SAV1) Focal deletion			ERBB2 amplifications, PRKCA/B translocations		
	FGFR2 translocations					
Clinical Features	Intra-neural invasion Moderate/poorly differentiated Poor prognosis (survival/recurrence)	Well differentiated Good prognosis		Papillary histology, Precursor lesions, dCCA	Poor prognosis	Good prognosis

Fig. 4. *Integrative classifications of iCCA and eCCA.* iCCAs can be classified into a *proliferation* and an *inflammation* class based on gene expression patterns. eCCA comprises four distinct subclasses: the *metabolic class*, the *proliferation class*, the *mesenchymal class*, and the *immune class*. The figure summarizes the main molecular features of each class.

to attenuated hepatocyte differentiation. These mutations can cooperate with *KRAS* mutations and drive expansion, development and metastatic progression of iCCA in mice.[48] The analysis on 52 iCCAs showed that *IDH*-mutated iCCAs present with hypermethylation, high number of chromosomal aberrations, and altered metabolic processes.[49]

In a phase III clinical trial using ivosidenib, an IDH1 inhibitor, progression-free survival improved with ivosidenib compared with placebo (median of 2·7 months vs 1·4 months).[50] Based on the success of this study, the FDA has recently granted approval to ivosidenib for patients with CCA harboring *IDH1* mutations. Further studies in a phase III clinical trials using ivosidenib to treat CCA patients with *IDH1* mutations show a 98% reduction of 2HG to levels resembling those of healthy patients.[51] On the contrary, results with IDH2 inhibitors have been discouraging. Finally, current clinical trials are using novel ways to treat IDH patients by inhibiting poly(ADP-Ribose) polymerase (PARP) with the drug olaparib. The treatment rationale is based on 2HG directly inhibiting homologous recombination and IDH mutants being more susceptible to PARP inhibition based on pre-clinical studies testing olaparib combined with radiotherapy in xenograft models.[52]

FGFR2 Fusions

FGFR2 gene fusions account for approximately 25% to 30% of all CCAs[45] and are most commonly found in iCCA than eCCA.[45,53] To date, more than 56 fusion partners[53–57] have been identified with the most common being *FGFR-B1CC1*.[58] Regardless of the specific gene involved, the fusion partner allows *FGFR2* to oligomerize in absence of FGF ligands, ultimately leading to activation of the respective FGFR kinase and enhanced cell proliferation.

Pemigatinib, a selective FGFR1-3 inhibitor, was the first-targeted therapy receiving accelerated FDA approval for CCA harboring *FGFR2* fusions or other rearrangements based on the results of a phase II clinical trial.[59] The 36% of patients with *FGFR2* fusions or rearrangements achieved an objective response, and 2.8% and 32.7% patients had confirmed complete responses and partial responses, respectively. Another inhibitor approved for CCA patients with *FGFR2* rearrangements is infigratinib, which is a selective adenosine triphosphate (ATP)-competitive inhibitor of FGFR.[60] Although the phase II showed promising results with 23.1% ORR and one patient with a confirmed CR, infigratinib ultimately did not provide a durable response.[60] In an evaluation of circulating free DNA

in three patients with acquired resistance to infigratinib, multiple de novo *FGFR2* point mutations were found at the time of progression that were not detected before treatment, with the point mutation, V564 F being present in all patients.[61] In in vitro studies introducing V564 F mutations in a BaF3 cell engineered to express *TEL-FGFR2* fusion protein, the cell line became resistant to infigratinib, highlighting the importance of de novo *FGFR2* mutations in the onset of acquired mechanism of resistance.[61]

Mismatch Repair Genes

ICIs are revolutionizing the clinical management of several cancers. Unfortunately, initial clinical results in unselected CCA populations treated with the anti-PD1 pembrolizumab have been disappointing, with only 6% to 13% of clinical responses[37] suggesting the critical need to identify biomarkers of response and resistance. ICIs are particularly effective in patients with mismatch repair (MMR) deficiency, with an observed clinical response in up to 40% of patients. MMR deficiency has been described in CCA, though it occurs only in small fraction of patients (~3%).[20] Interestingly, in four CCA patients with high MSI receiving pembrolizumab, one exhibited complete response, whereas the remaining three showed stable disease.[62]

EPIGENETICS OF CHOLANGIOCARCINOMA

Studies in epigenetic alterations in cancer have shown the limitations of the clonal genetic model in explaining CCA tumorigenesis, progression, and metastasis. Whole-exome and whole-genome sequencing data of CCA have shown mutations in epigenetic regulators, including *IDH1/2*, *AT-Rich interaction domain 1A* (*ARID1A*), *BRCA1 associated protein-1* (*BAP1*), and *polybromo-1* (*PBRM1*).[20] Methylation of at least one tumor suppressor genes has been described in 85% of all CCA.[63] The top four tumor suppressors that were methylated include *Ras association domain-containing protein 1* (*RASSF1A*), *cyclin-dependent kinase 4 inhibitor B* (*p15INK4b*), *cyclin-dependent kinase inhibitor 2A* (*p16INK4a*), and *adenomatous polyposis coli* (*APC*). Interestingly, *RASSF1A* methylation is more common in eCCA (83% vs 47%), whereas *GSTP* methylation is more common in iCCA (31% vs 6%).[64] Overall, hypermethylation is characteristic of iCCA; hypermethylated sites have been specifically found in transcription factors and high mobility group (HMG) box domain binding, although hypomethylation mostly occurs in gene bodies, heterochromatic, and quiescent regions.[49]

Targeting epigenetic pathway has introduced a novel mode of therapy for CCA. A study looking into targeting both G9a, a histone methyltransferase, and DNA methyltransferase 1 (DNMT1) by using the dual-inhibitor CM272, has shown promise in in vitro and in vivo models.[65]

SUMMARY

Over the years, clinical trials testing molecular therapies in unselected CCA populations have been discouraging. The recent clinical success achieved with IDH and FGFR inhibitors suggest that, to improve patient prognosis, the design of more personalized treatments—tailored to the molecular characteristics of the tumor—is becoming critical. Nonetheless, given the ability of the tumor and its surrounding stroma to overcome blockade of these oncogenic signaling, a deeper understanding of the TME interactions is desperately needed. Future efforts should take advantage of emerging single-cell technologies to further clarify the pathogenesis of CCA and understand how genetic and epigenetic features of the tumor may influence the immunobiology of this disease and vice versa. This information will be key in designing more effective combination strategies targeting both the tumor and its surrounding microenvironment.

CLINICS CARE POINTS

- Most of the patients with cholangiocarcinoma (CCA) are diagnosed at advanced stage when palliative chemotherapy represents the first-line therapy.

- The IDH1 inhibitor ivosidenib has recently received FDA approval for previously treated patients with CCA harboring *IDH1* mutation.

- The FGFR inhibitors, pemigatinib, and infigratinib have received accelerated FDA approval for previously treated patients with CCA harboring an FGFR2 rearrangement.

- The recent successes with IDH1 and FGFR inhibitors suggest that genomic profiling of the tumor should be recommend to all patients with advanced CCA.

DISCLOSURE

The authors have nothing to disclose.

REFERENCES

1. Banales JM, Marin JJG, Lamarca A, et al. Cholangiocarcinoma 2020: the next horizon in mechanisms and management. Nat Rev Gastroenterol Hepatol 2020;17(9):557–88.
2. Moeini A, Haber PK, Sia D. Cell of origin in biliary tract cancers and clinical implications. JHEP Rep 2021;3(2):100226.
3. Khan SA, Tavolari S, Brandi G. Cholangiocarcinoma: epidemiology and risk factors. Liver Int 2019;39(Suppl 1):19–31.
4. Banales JM, Cardinale V, Carpino G, et al. Expert consensus document: Cholangiocarcinoma: current knowledge and future perspectives consensus statement from the European Network for the Study of Cholangiocarcinoma (ENS-CCA). Nat Rev Gastroenterol Hepatol 2016;13(5):261–80.
5. Sia D, Villanueva A, Friedman SL, et al. Liver Cancer Cell of Origin, Molecular Class, and Effects on Patient Prognosis. Gastroenterology 2017;152(4):745–61.
6. Kumari N, Dwarakanath BS, Das A, et al. Role of interleukin-6 in cancer progression and therapeutic resistance. Tumour Biol 2016;37(9):11553–72.
7. Kobayashi S, Werneburg NW, Bronk SF, et al. Interleukin-6 contributes to Mcl-1 up-regulation and TRAIL resistance via an Akt-signaling pathway in cholangiocarcinoma cells. Gastroenterology 2005;128(7):2054–65.
8. Cheon YK, Cho YD, Moon JH, et al. Diagnostic utility of interleukin-6 (IL-6) for primary bile duct cancer and changes in serum IL-6 levels following photodynamic therapy. Am J Gastroenterol 2007;102(10):2164–70.
9. Nguyen MLT, Bui KC, Scholta T, et al. Targeting interleukin 6 signaling by monoclonal antibody siltuximab on cholangiocarcinoma. J Gastroenterol Hepatol 2021;36(5):1334–45.
10. Zong Y, Panikkar A, Xu J, et al. Notch signaling controls liver development by regulating biliary differentiation. Development 2009;136(10):1727–39.
11. Valizadeh A, Sayadmanesh A, Asemi Z, et al. Regulatory Roles of the Notch Signaling Pathway in Liver Repair and Regeneration: A Novel Therapeutic Target. Curr Med Chem 2021;28(41):8608–26.
12. O'Rourke CJ, Matter MS, Nepal C, et al. Identification of a Pan-Gamma-Secretase Inhibitor Response Signature for Notch-Driven Cholangiocarcinoma. Hepatology 2020;71(1):196–213.
13. Aoki S, Mizuma M, Takahashi Y, et al. Aberrant activation of Notch signaling in extrahepatic cholangiocarcinoma: clinicopathological features and therapeutic potential for cancer stem cell-like properties. BMC Cancer 2016;16(1):854.
14. Lu X, Peng B, Chen G, et al. YAP Accelerates Notch-Driven Cholangiocarcinogenesis via mTORC1 in Mice. Am J Pathol 2021;191(9):1651–67.

15. Pan D. The hippo signaling pathway in development and cancer. Dev Cell 2010;19(4):491–505.

16. Marti P, Stein C, Blumer T, et al. YAP promotes proliferation, chemoresistance, and angiogenesis in human cholangiocarcinoma through TEAD transcription factors. Hepatology 2015;62(5): 1497–510.

17. Ma W, Han C, Zhang J, et al. The Histone Methyltransferase G9a Promotes Cholangiocarcinogenesis Through Regulation of the Hippo Pathway Kinase LATS2 and YAP Signaling Pathway. Hepatology 2020;72(4):1283–97.

18. Moya IM, Castaldo SA, Van den Mooter L, et al. Peritumoral activation of the Hippo pathway effectors YAP and TAZ suppresses liver cancer in mice. Science 2019;366(6468):1029–34.

19. Wang W, Smits R, Hao H, et al. Wnt/β-Catenin Signaling in Liver Cancers. Cancers (Basel) 2019; 11(7). https://doi.org/10.3390/cancers11070926.

20. Haber PK, Sia D. Translating cancer genomics for precision oncology in biliary tract cancers. Discov Med 2019;28(155):255–65.

21. Zheng Y, Zhou C, Yu XX, et al. Osteopontin promotes metastasis of intrahepatic cholangiocarcinoma through recruiting MAPK1 and mediating Ser675 phosphorylation of β-Catenin. Cell Death Dis 2018;9(2):179.

22. Jing CY, Fu YP, Zhou C, et al. Hepatic stellate cells promote intrahepatic cholangiocarcinoma progression via NR4A2/osteopontin/Wnt signaling axis. Oncogene 2021;40(16):2910–22.

23. Krishnamurthy N, Kurzrock R. Targeting the Wnt/beta-catenin pathway in cancer: Update on effectors and inhibitors. Cancer Treat Rev 2018;62: 50–60.

24. Messersmith WA, Shapiro GI, Cleary JM, et al. A Phase I, dose-finding study in patients with advanced solid malignancies of the oral γ-secretase inhibitor PF-03084014. Clin Cancer Res 2015;21(1): 60–7.

25. Moehler M, Maderer A, Ehrlich A, et al. Safety and efficacy of afatinib as add-on to standard therapy of gemcitabine/cisplatin in chemotherapy-naive patients with advanced biliary tract cancer: an open-label, phase I trial with an extensive biomarker program. BMC Cancer 2019;19(1):55.

26. Chiang NJ, Hsu C, Chen JS, et al. Expression levels of ROS1/ALK/c-MET and therapeutic efficacy of cetuximab plus chemotherapy in advanced biliary tract cancer. Sci Rep 2016;6:25369.

27. Ueno M, Ikeda M, Sasaki T, et al. Phase 2 study of lenvatinib monotherapy as second-line treatment in unresectable biliary tract cancer: primary analysis results. BMC Cancer 2020;20(1):1105.

28. Iyer RV, Pokuri VK, Groman A, et al. A Multicenter Phase II Study of Gemcitabine, Capecitabine, and Bevacizumab for Locally Advanced or Metastatic Biliary Tract Cancer. Am J Clin Oncol 2018;41(7): 649–55.

29. Torrens L, Montironi C, Puigvehí M, et al. Immunomodulatory effects of lenvatinib plus anti-PD1 in mice and rationale for patient enrichment in hepatocellular carcinoma. Hepatology 2021. https://doi.org/10.1002/hep.32023.

30. Chuaysri C, Thuwajit P, Paupairoj A, et al. Alpha-smooth muscle actin-positive fibroblasts promote biliary cell proliferation and correlate with poor survival in cholangiocarcinoma. Oncol Rep 2009; 21(4):957–69.

31. Tamma R, Annese T, Ruggieri S, et al. Inflammatory cells infiltrate and angiogenesis in locally advanced and metastatic cholangiocarcinoma. Eur J Clin Invest 2019;49(5):e13087.

32. Affo S, Nair A, Brundu F, et al. Promotion of cholangiocarcinoma growth by diverse cancer-associated fibroblast subpopulations. Cancer Cell 2021;39(6): 866–82.e11.

33. Zhang M, Yang H, Wan L, et al. Single-cell transcriptomic architecture and intercellular crosstalk of human intrahepatic cholangiocarcinoma. J Hepatol 2020;73(5):1118–30.

34. Atanasov G, Hau HM, Dietel C, et al. Prognostic significance of macrophage invasion in hilar cholangiocarcinoma. BMC Cancer 2015;15:790.

35. Hasita H, Komohara Y, Okabe H, et al. Significance of alternatively activated macrophages in patients with intrahepatic cholangiocarcinoma. Cancer Sci 2010;101(8):1913–9.

36. Loeuillard E, Conboy CB, Gores GJ, et al. Immunobiology of cholangiocarcinoma. JHEP Rep 2019; 1(4):297–311.

37. Piha-Paul SA, Oh DY, Ueno M, et al. Efficacy and safety of pembrolizumab for the treatment of advanced biliary cancer: Results from the KEYNOTE-158 and KEYNOTE-028 studies. Int J Cancer 2020;147(8):2190–8.

38. Sia D, Hoshida Y, Villanueva A, et al. Integrative molecular analysis of intrahepatic cholangiocarcinoma reveals 2 classes that have different outcomes. Gastroenterology 2013;144(4):829–40.

39. Andersen JB, Spee B, Blechacz BR, et al. Genomic and genetic characterization of cholangiocarcinoma identifies therapeutic targets for tyrosine kinase inhibitors. Gastroenterology 2012;142(4).

40. Oishi N, Kumar MR, Roessler S, et al. Transcriptomic profiling reveals hepatic stem-like gene signatures and interplay of miR-200c and epithelial-mesenchymal transition in intrahepatic cholangiocarcinoma. Hepatology 2012;56(5):1792–803.

41. Montal R, Sia D, Montironi C, et al. Molecular classification and therapeutic targets in extrahepatic cholangiocarcinoma. J Hepatol 2020;73(2):315–27.

42. Job S, Rapoud D, Dos Santos A, et al. Identification of Four Immune Subtypes Characterized by Distinct

Composition and Functions of Tumor Microenvironment in Intrahepatic Cholangiocarcinoma. Hepatology 2020;72(3):965–81.

43. Martin-Serrano MA, Kepecs B, Torres-Martin M, et al. Novel microenvironment-based classification of intrahepatic cholangiocarcinoma with therapeutic implications. Gut 2022. https://doi.org/10.1136/gutjnl-2021-326514.

44. Zhuang X, Xiao YP, Tan LH, et al. Efficacy and safety of chemotherapy with or without targeted therapy in biliary tract cancer: A meta-analysis of 7 randomized controlled trials. J Huazhong Univ Sci Technolog Med Sci 2017;37(2):172–8.

45. Lowery MA, Ptashkin R, Jordan E, et al. Comprehensive Molecular Profiling of Intrahepatic and Extrahepatic Cholangiocarcinomas: Potential Targets for Intervention. Clin Cancer Res 2018;24(17):4154–61.

46. Chen Y, Chi P. Basket trial of TRK inhibitors demonstrates efficacy in TRK fusion-positive cancers. J Hematol Oncol 2018;11(1):78.

47. Salati M, Caputo F, Baldessari C, et al. IDH Signalling Pathway in Cholangiocarcinoma: From Biological Rationale to Therapeutic Targeting. Cancers (Basel) 2020;12(11). https://doi.org/10.3390/cancers12113310.

48. Saha SK, Parachoniak CA, Ghanta KS, et al. Mutant IDH inhibits HNF-4α to block hepatocyte differentiation and promote biliary cancer. Nature 2014;513(7516):110–4. https://doi.org/10.1038/nature13441.

49. Goeppert B, Toth R, Singer S, et al. Integrative Analysis Defines Distinct Prognostic Subgroups of Intrahepatic Cholangiocarcinoma. Hepatology 2019;69(5):2091–106. https://doi.org/10.1002/hep.30493.

50. Abou-Alfa GK, Macarulla T, Javle MM, et al. Ivosidenib in IDH1-mutant, chemotherapy-refractory cholangiocarcinoma (ClarIDHy): a multicentre, randomised, double-blind, placebo-controlled, phase 3 study. The Lancet Oncol 2020;21(6):796–807. https://doi.org/10.1016/s1470-2045(20)30157-1.

51. Fan B, Mellinghoff IK, Wen PY, et al. Clinical pharmacokinetics and pharmacodynamics of ivosidenib, an oral, targeted inhibitor of mutant IDH1, in patients with advanced solid tumors. Invest New Drugs 2020;38(2):433–44. https://doi.org/10.1007/s10637-019-00771-x.

52. Wang Y, Wild AT, Turcan S, et al. Targeting therapeutic vulnerabilities with PARP inhibition and radiation in IDH-mutant gliomas and cholangiocarcinomas. Sci Adv 2020;6(17):eaaz3221.

53. Arai Y, Totoki Y, Hosoda F, et al. Fibroblast growth factor receptor 2 tyrosine kinase fusions define a unique molecular subtype of cholangiocarcinoma. Hepatology 2014;59(4):1427–34.

54. Borad MJ, Champion MD, Egan JB, et al. Integrated genomic characterization reveals novel, therapeutically relevant drug targets in FGFR and EGFR pathways in sporadic intrahepatic cholangiocarcinoma. Plos Genet 2014;10(2):e1004135.

55. Nakamura H, Arai Y, Totoki Y, et al. Genomic spectra of biliary tract cancer. Nat Genet 2015;47(9):1003–10.

56. Sia D, Losic B, Moeini A, et al. Massive parallel sequencing uncovers actionable FGFR2–PPHLN1 fusion and ARAF mutations in intrahepatic cholangiocarcinoma. Nat Commun 2015;6(1):6087.

57. Wu YM, Su F, Kalyana-Sundaram S, et al. Identification of targetable FGFR gene fusions in diverse cancers. Cancer Discov 2013;3(6):636–47.

58. Silverman IM, Hollebecque A, Friboulet L, et al. Clinicogenomic Analysis of FGFR2-Rearranged Cholangiocarcinoma Identifies Correlates of Response and Mechanisms of Resistance to Pemigatinib. Cancer Discov 2021;11(2):326–39.

59. Liu PCC, Koblish H, Wu L, et al. INCB054828 (pemigatinib), a potent and selective inhibitor of fibroblast growth factor receptors 1, 2, and 3, displays activity against genetically defined tumor models. PLOS ONE 2020;15(4):e0231877.

60. Javle M, Roychowdhury S, Kelley RK, et al. Infigratinib (BGJ398) in previously treated patients with advanced or metastatic cholangiocarcinoma with FGFR2 fusions or rearrangements: mature results from a multicentre, open-label, single-arm, phase 2 study. Lancet Gastroenterol Hepatol 2021. https://doi.org/10.1016/s2468-1253(21)00196-5.

61. Goyal L, Saha SK, Liu LY, et al. Polyclonal Secondary FGFR2 Mutations Drive Acquired Resistance to FGFR Inhibition in Patients with FGFR2 Fusion–Positive Cholangiocarcinoma. Cancer Discov 2017;7(3):252–63.

62. Le DT, Durham JN, Smith KN, et al. Mismatch repair deficiency predicts response of solid tumors to PD-1 blockade. Science 2017;357(6349):409–13.

63. Goeppert B, Konermann C, Schmidt CR, et al. Global alterations of DNA methylation in cholangiocarcinoma target the Wnt signaling pathway. Hepatology 2014;59(2):544–54.

64. Yang B, House MG, Guo M, et al. Promoter methylation profiles of tumor suppressor genes in intrahepatic and extrahepatic cholangiocarcinoma. Mod Pathol 2005;18(3):412–20.

65. Colyn L, Bárcena-Varela M, Álvarez-Sola G, et al. Dual Targeting of G9a and DNA Methyltransferase-1 for the Treatment of Experimental Cholangiocarcinoma. Hepatology 2021;73(6):2380–96.

66. Valle JW, Lamarca A, Goyal L, et al. New Horizons for Precision Medicine in Biliary Tract Cancers. Cancer Discov 2017;7(9):943–62.

Prognostic and Predictive Biomarkers for Pancreatic Neuroendocrine Tumors

Wenzel M. Hackeng, MD, PhD[a], Hussein A. Assi, MD[b],
Florine H.M. Westerbeke, BSc (Med)[a],
Lodewijk A.A. Brosens, MD, PhD[a],
Christopher M. Heaphy, PhD[c,d,*]

KEYWORDS

• Alternative lengthening of telomeres • ARX • ATRX • DAXX • Epigenetics • PDX1 • Prognosis

---

Key points

- Current prognostic indicators for pancreatic neuroendocrine tumors (PanNETs) are imperfect predictors of outcome, thus novel prognostic biomarkers are needed to *accurately predict prognosis and potential response to targeted therapies*.

- Numerous independent studies have validated alternative lengthening of telomeres and ATRX/DAXX loss as poor prognostic biomarkers in primary PanNETs, and importantly, even in small (<2 cm) tumors.

- PanNET subtypes based on epigenetic profiling tend to resemble α-cells or β-cells and differ in mutational signatures, specific chromosomal alterations, and clinical outcomes.

- Future prospective studies combining genetic and epigenetic profiling are warranted and may lead to clinically useful information that will help optimize and personalize patient outcomes.

ABSTRACT

Pancreatic neuroendocrine tumors (PanNETs) represent a clinically challenging disease because these tumors vary in clinical presentation, natural history, and prognosis. Novel prognostic biomarkers are needed to improve patient stratification and treatment options. Several putative prognostic and/or predictive biomarkers (eg, alternative lengthening of telomeres, alpha-thalassemia/mental retardation, X linked (ATRX)/Death Domain Associated Protein (DAXX) loss) have been independently validated. Additionally, recent transcriptomic and epigenetic studies focusing on endocrine differentiation have identified PanNET subtypes that display similarities to either α-cells or β-cells and differ in clinical outcomes. Thus, future prospective studies that incorporate genomic and epigenetic biomarkers are warranted and have translational potential for individualized therapeutic and surveillance strategies.

INTRODUCTION

Neuroendocrine neoplasms are a diverse group of neoplasms that originate from cells in the diffuse neuroendocrine system. These unique neoplasms can arise in almost every organ in the body;

---

[a] Department of Pathology, University Medical Center Utrecht, Utrecht University, Heidelberglaan 100, 3584 CX Utrecht, the Netherlands; [b] Department of Medicine, Boston University School of Medicine, 820 Harrison Avenue, FGH 2011, Boston, MA 02118, USA; [c] Department of Medicine, Boston University School of Medicine, 650 Albany Street, Room 444, Boston, MA 02118, USA; [d] Department of Pathology & Laboratory Medicine, Boston University School of Medicine, 650 Albany Street, Room 444, Boston, MA 02118, USA
* Corresponding author. Department of Medicine, Boston University School of Medicine, 650 Albany Street, Room 444, Boston, MA 02118.
E-mail address: heaphyc@bu.edu

Table 1
Hereditary syndromes associated with pancreatic neuroendocrine tumors

Hereditary Syndrome	Prevalence (per 100,000)	Affected Gene	Prevalence of PanNETs	Type of PanNET
Multiple endocrine neoplasia type 1 (MEN1)	1–10	MEN1	30%–80%	Functional and nonfunctional
von Hippel-Lindau syndrome (VHL)	2–3	VHL	8%–17%	Nonfunctional
Neurofibromatosis 1	20–50	NF1	0%–10%	Somatostatinomas (often duodenal)
Tuberous sclerosis complex (TSC)	10	TSC1 or TSC2	0%–1%	Functional and nonfunctional
Familial insulinomatosis		MAFA		Insulinomas
Glucagon cell hyperplasia and neoplasia		GCGR		Glucagonomas

Abbreviation: GCGR, Glucagon Receptor; MAFA, MAF BZIP Transcription Factor A; NF1, Neurofibromin 1; PanNET, pancreatic neuroendocrine tumor; TSC1, Tuberous sclerosis 1; TSC2, Tuberous sclerosis 2.

however, the gastrointestinal tract, pancreas, and lungs are the most common sites of origin.[1] Pancreatic neuroendocrine neoplasms (PanNENs) are classified based on their histology and are subdivided into well-differentiated pancreatic neuroendocrine tumors (PanNETs) and poorly differentiated neuroendocrine carcinomas (PanNECs). PanNECs are rare, aggressive malignancies, and their genomic alteration profiles dramatically differ compared with PanNETs.[2] In this review, we will specifically focus on PanNETs.

Representing up to 10% of all tumors arising from the pancreas, PanNETs are the second most common solid pancreatic tumor, after pancreatic ductal adenocarcinoma.[3,4] The incidence of PanNETs is less than 1 per 100,000 persons per year, although the incidence is increasing due to the improved and increased use of medical imaging.[1,4] PanNETs are clinically classified into either nonfunctional or functional tumors. Nonfunctional PanNETs (NF-PanNETs) account for 60% to 90% of all PanNETs.[1,5] NF-PanNETs either do not produce active hormones or peptides, or the production does not lead to any related clinical symptoms.[5] Thus, these tumors are regularly asymptomatic and, therefore, often only diagnosed incidentally on imaging. Alternatively, they can be diagnosed because of symptoms caused by mass effect of the primary tumor or distant metastases.[6,7] In contrast, functional PanNETs are characterized by their inappropriate active (over) production of hormones or peptides. The clinical symptoms of a functional PanNET depend on the type of hormone or peptide, which is produced by the tumor; for instance, insulin, gastrin, glucagon,

vasoactive intestinal peptide, and somatostatin. Due to the presence of such a clinical syndrome, functional PanNETs are mostly diagnosed at a younger age than NF-PanNETs.[2,6] Functional PanNETs are diagnosed at a mean age of 55 years, whereas patients with NF-PanNETs have a mean of 59 years at time of diagnosis.[4] The most common types of functional PanNETs are the insulin-secreting PanNETs, or insulinomas, followed by gastrin-secreting PanNETs, or gastrinomas.[1,2,5–8] However, gastrinomas are more often from duodenal origin rather than pancreatic origin.[1,8] Patients with insulinomas tend to have increased levels of insulin and associated symptoms. Typically, these patients present with the "Whipple's triad"; consisting of low plasma levels of glucose, symptoms and signs of hypoglycemia, and resolution of symptoms after correction of the hypoglycemia.[1,2,6–9] Patients with gastrinomas, also called Zollinger-Ellison syndrome, suffer from symptoms related to high levels of serum gastrin. This leads to increased production of gastric acid causing refractory peptic ulcer disease in the stomach and duodenum, gastroesophageal reflux, and sometimes secretory diarrhea.[5,6,8]

PanNETs can arise as part of different autosomal dominantly inherited syndromes. The main syndrome associated with PanNETs is multiple endocrine neoplasia type 1 (MEN1) syndrome.[10–13] MEN1 patients tend to develop multiple primary tumors in affected tissues, including the parathyroid glands, pancreas, and duodenum. PanNETs arise in approximately 30% to 80% of all MEN1 patients.[13–15] Age at diagnosis of PanNETs is generally much younger in MEN1 patients compared with sporadic cases: 10 to 50 years versus 50 to 80 years, respectively.[14–16] PanNETs are usually nonfunctional in MEN1 patients, although functional PanNETs can occur. For example, gastrinomas are the most common type of functional enteropancreatic neuroendocrine tumors in this patient population, yet they most often occur primarily in the duodenum. Thus, insulinomas are the most common type of functional PanNETs in MEN1 patients, representing 10% to 30% of all PanNETs in this group.[14,15] In addition, patients with Von Hippel-Lindau Tumor Suppressor (VHL), neurofibromatosis 1, and tuberous sclerosis complex (TSC), are at increased risk of developing PanNETs (Table 1).[10–13,17] For example, the prevalence of PanNETs in patients with VHL ranges from 8% to 17%, and the tumors are most often nonfunctional.[10–13,16] In addition to the hereditary syndromes mentioned above, familial insulinomatosis and glucagon cell hyperplasia and neoplasia are 2 virtually unknown and extremely rare hereditary syndromes that can cause specific types of PanNETs (see Table 1).[18,19]

Prognosis of PanNETs is currently mainly determined by the World Health Organization (WHO) grade. Recent genetic and epigenetic studies have revealed novel subtypes and potential new prognostic biomarkers.[1,20] Increasing the use of prognostic biomarkers may improve the diagnostic work-up and stratification and management of patients with PanNETs. Current prognostic biomarkers, as well as novel insights from recent genetic and epigenetic studies, will be discussed in this review.

ESTABLISHED PROGNOSTIC BIOMARKERS

The heterogeneity in PanNETs at the pathologic level translates into a wide spectrum of varying clinical behaviors and treatment responses. Several prognostic and predictive factors have been investigated in retrospective studies, including clinical, pathologic, and molecular markers.[21] Nevertheless, there remains a paucity in validated independent prognostic PanNET biomarkers. The WHO grading classification along with the eighth edition American Joint Committee on Cancer (AJCC) Tumor-Node-Metastasis (TNM) staging system are the most widely used prognostic parameters in clinical practice.[22] The WHO grading classification is based on morphology, as measured by the degree of differentiation, and cellular proliferation, as measured by the Ki-67 index and mitotic count. As shown in Table 2, this grading classification was updated in 2017 to reflect the distinction between well-differentiated G3 PanNETs and poorly differentiated G3 PanNECs, and more recently in 2019, with the addition of the mixed neuroendocrine–nonneuroendocrine neoplasms category.[23,24] A recent study of 480 patients with PanNETs or PanNECs supports the prognostic stratification by WHO grade, with statistically significant overall survival (OS) difference between all groups in multivariate analyses.[25] Poorly differentiated PanNECs have an approximate 4.5-fold increase in the risk of death compared with well-differentiated PanNETs, highlighting the prognostic importance of cellular morphology.[25] Ki-67 index has a high interinstitutional reliability as a proliferative marker and has been shown in a large systematic review of 22 studies to be a significant prognostic marker for disease-free survival (DFS) and OS.[26,27] Similarly, mitotic count has also been shown to be a prognostic marker for DFS and OS on multivariate analysis.[28] Interestingly, studies have reported a discordance rate of 17% to 37% between Ki-67 and mitotic count.[28,29] In discordant cases, although both Ki-67 and mitotic

Table 2
World Health Organization 2019 classification for gastroenteropancreatic neuroendocrine neoplasms

Terminology	Differentiation	Grade	Mitotic Count (Mitoses/2 mm^3)	Ki-67 Index (%)
NET, G1	Well differentiated	Low	<2	<3
NET, G2	Well differentiated	Intermediate	2–20	3–20
NET, G3	Well differentiated	High	>20	>20
NEC, small cell type	Poorly differentiated	High	>20	>20
NEC, large cell type	Poorly differentiated	High	>20	>20
MiNEN	Usually poorly differentiated	Usually high	Variable	Variable

Abbreviations: G, World Health Organization grade; MiNEN, mixed neuroendocrine-nonneuroendocrine neoplasms; NEC, neuroendocrine carcinoma; NEN, neuroendocrine neoplasm; NET, neuroendocrine tumor; WHO, World Health Organization.

rate should be reported, the method leading to the highest grade determines the grade of the tumor.[1] A study of 297 patients with PanNETs showed that the survival among discordant mitotic grade 1 (G1) tumors is lower than concordant G1 tumors but similar to concordant grade 2 (G2) tumors.[29] Therefore, it is crucial to incorporate both Ki-67 and mitotic count to accurately define tumor grade, and thereby prognosis.

Somatostatin receptor 2 (SSTR-2) expression by immunohistochemistry was also found to be an independent prognostic marker.[30,31] However, although SSTR-2 positivity by imaging is a predictive marker for response to peptide receptor radionuclide therapy (PRRT), this has not been shown to be the case for SSTR-2 immunohistochemistry.[30] Clinically, disease stage dictates both prognosis and treatment strategies. Although the overall AJCC TNM stage has been validated as a clinical prognostic factor for DFS and OS,[32] the prognostic value of tumor size remains controversial. Although some studies show that tumor size is associated with worse survival outcome,[33,34] large database studies and meta-analyses failed to confirm tumor size as an independent prognostic factor.[35,36] Nevertheless, tumor size is an important factor to consider in the management of Pan-NETs based on consensus guidelines,[37,38] as discussed below.

GENERAL PRINCIPLES OF CLINICAL MANAGEMENT AND PROGNOSIS

The management of localized or locoregional Pan-NETs generally involves surgical resection, especially in symptomatic or functional tumors.[37,38] However, many low-grade PanNETs behave indolently, and thus active surveillance has been suggested as an alternative management strategy. The challenge lies in determining the factors that would effectively predict indolent behavior. A matched case-control study of patients with incidental, sporadic, small (<3 cm) PanNETs showed that none of the patients in the observation group developed disease recurrence.[39] Two retrospective studies showed that even small NF-PanNETs (<2 cm) that underwent surgical resection had a rate of recurrence around 10%.[40,41] Given the conflicting results and lack of prospective data, the optimal tumor size cutoff is still debated. Nevertheless, most consensus guidelines advocate for active surveillance for small (<1–2 cm), nonfunctional, asymptomatic low-grade Pan-NETs.[37,38] The Asymptomatic Small Pancreatic Endocrine Neoplasms (ASPEN) study, a prospective cohort study designed to evaluate active

surveillance compared with surgical resection in asymptomatic NF-PanNETs 2 cm or lesser, is currently open for recruitment.[42]

Surgical resection and liver-directed therapy (LDT) are increasingly being incorporated in the management of metastatic PanNETs, especially in patients with symptomatic disease, as well as limited disease burden confined to the liver. Early data showed that patients undergoing cytoreductive surgery, whether palliative or curative intent, had a prolonged OS compared with historical controls.[43] Although an initial arbitrary threshold of greater than 90% debulking was used as a threshold, a recent study in which a 70% threshold was used on 42 patients with PanNETs showed no difference in outcome based on percentage debulked (70%–89% vs 90%–99% vs 100%), providing evidence that the cytoreduction threshold can ultimately be reduced to 70%.[43] Another series, including 41 patients with a Pan-NET, found no difference in DFS or OS with respect to the number of liver lesions treated with resection or LDT.[43] Consistent with previous studies, less than 70% cytoreduction was associated with significantly inferior OS compared with those who underwent greater than 70% cytoreduction (38 vs 134 months, respectively).[44] Because all studies are retrospective in nature and suffer from potential selection bias, this remains a controversial issue.

The choice of systemic therapy in PanNETs largely depends on the tumor grade and differentiation. Low-grade PanNETs are typically treated with somatostatin analogs (SSAs) as first-line therapy. The SSA Lanreotide is associated with a higher DFS rate at 24 months compared with placebo in patients with treatment-naïve G1 or G2 gastroenteropancreatic NETs (65% vs 33%).[45] Targeted therapy (everolimus or sunitinib) or PRRT (for SSTR-positive disease only) are approved for use in patients with PanNETs after disease progression on an SSA. The mTOR inhibitor, everolimus, is associated with a superior median progression-free survival (PFS) compared with placebo in advanced PanNETs (11 vs 4.6 months), as well as a higher response rate (5% vs 2%, respectively).[46] Sunitinib, a tyrosine kinase inhibitor, also showed a superior median PFS compared with placebo (11.4 vs 5.5 months) and a higher response rate (9.3% vs 0%, respectively).[47] In both studies, no OS benefit was detected due to crossover. PRRT is approved for SSTR-positive G1/G2 NETs who have progressed on an SSA, with updated survival data published in 2021, showing continued statistically significant improvement in PFS compared with a high-dose SSA (Hazard ratio (HR) 0.18) and a trend toward median OS improvement of nearly 12 months.[48] The exact sequence of therapy has yet to be defined, with ongoing clinical trials, such as the COMPETE trial, attempting to answer such questions (https://clinicaltrials.gov/ct2/show/NCT03049189). However, progressive G1/G2 PanNETs, G3 PanNETs, and PanNECs benefit from cytotoxic chemotherapy.[37] Temozolomide, alone or in combination with Capecitabine, is associated with a response rate of 34% and 51%, respectively, in patients with advanced PanNETs.[49] Although beyond the scope of this review, other cytotoxic chemotherapy options also include 5-fluorouracil-based therapy and platinum-based therapy for PanNECs.[50,51]

GENETIC ALTERATIONS WITH PROGNOSTIC AND/OR PREDICTIVE POTENTIAL

A decade ago, our knowledge of the genetics underlying the initiation and progression of PanNETs was limited. However, advances in sequencing technologies revealed the molecular alterations underpinning PanNET development, as well as identified several putative prognostic and/or predictive biomarkers. Although numerous studies contributed to these findings, 2 seminal studies advanced the field forward, including a whole-exome study of 68 cases (10 in the discovery cohort and 58 in the validation cohort)[52] and a whole-genome and RNA-sequencing study of 160 cases (98 in the discovery cohort and 62 in the validation cohort).[53] Although primary and metastatic cases were included, these studies mostly consisted of sporadic, nonfunctional, well-differentiated G1/G2 PanNETs. As previously described by other targeted sequencing studies, frequent mutations in MEN1, which encodes for the tumor suppressor menin,[54] were identified in 37% to 44% of cases, although genomic or chromosomal alterations in MEN1 likely occur in most of PanNETs.[53]

In addition to MEN1 mutations, recurrent inactivating mutations occur in the ATRX and DAXX genes, which encode a chromatin-remodeling complex.[52] As shown in **Fig. 1**, these loss-of-function mutations usually lead to loss of nuclear protein expression; therefore, immunohistochemistry has been extensively used as a surrogate for the presence of inactivating mutations.[52,55–57] Importantly, these somatic mutations are mutually exclusive and strongly correlate with the alternative lengthening of telomeres (ALT), a telomerase-independent telomere maintenance mechanism.[58,59] Forming a histone chaperone complex, ATRX/DAXX functions to deposit the histone variant H3.3 in heterochromatic regions of chromosomes containing highly repetitive elements, in particular pericentromeric and telomeric regions.[60] Due to telomere-specific chromatin alterations leading to telomere deprotection, ALT-positive PanNETs maintain telomere lengths through a homology-directed DNA repair mechanism, similar to break-induced repair, thereby resulting in rampant DNA damage and replicative stress.[61] Interestingly, ATRX and DAXX mutations

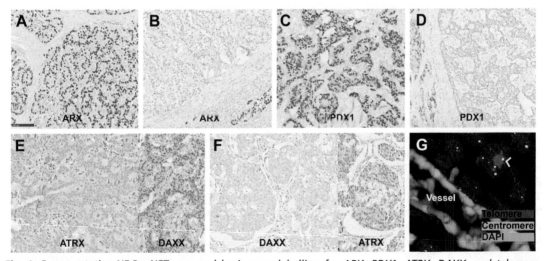

Fig. 1. Representative NF-PanNETs assessed by immunolabelling for ARX, PDX1, ATRX, DAXX, and telomere-specific fluorescence in situ hybridization for ALT. (*A*) Positive ARX expression; (*B*) absent ARX expression with positive Islet control; (*C*) positive PDX1 expression; (*D*) absent PDX1 expression with normal acinar control; (*E*) absent ATRX expression with positive stromal controls, positive DAXX in the same area; (*F*) absent DAXX expression with positive stromal controls, positive ATRX in the same area; and (*G*) ultrabright telomeric FISH signals in tumor nuclei indicative of ALT near an autofluorescent vessel.

have not been identified in microadenomas, the precursor to PanNETs, thereby suggesting these mutations do not directly initiate tumorigenesis but rather promote tumor development.[62,63] Importantly, the presence of ALT and/or alterations in ATRX/DAXX (either by mutation or nuclear protein loss) have been identified and independently validated as robust prognostic biomarkers in large cohorts of primary Pan-NETs.[53,55–57,64–70] These biomarkers are independently associated with aggressive clinico-pathologic behavior and reduced recurrence-free survival, thereby emphasizing the notable role these alterations play in promoting metastatic disease. Highlighting these findings, a recent international, multi-institutional cohort study of more than 560 nonsyndromic/NF-PanNETs without distant metastases at surgical resection demonstrated that ALT (and ATRX/DAXX protein loss) was strongly associated with numerous adverse prognostic features, most notably with the presence of metachronous distant metastases/recurrences (see Fig. 1).[41] Of importance for identifying biomarkers that may be used in the setting of surveillance of small tumors, the study included subgroup analyses of 196 cases that were 2.0 cm or lesser in size without regional lymph node metastases. Similar to the full cohort analysis, ALT and ATRX/DAXX loss were independent prognostic biomarkers for decreased recurrence-free survival in these small tumors.[41] Based on these data, several groups have now independently advocated that ALT and ATRX/DAXX loss should be implemented into clinical practice to identify patients with localized NF-PanNETs that are at a higher risk of recurrence.[71,72]

Additionally, recurrent somatic mutations in primary PanNETs occur to varying degrees in pathways involving mTOR signaling, DNA damage repair, and chromatin remodeling. In general, mutations in these pathways are enriched in patients with locally advanced or metastatic disease.[73–75] Approximately 15% of PanNETs have somatic mutations in genes involved in the mTOR pathway, including TSC1/TSC2, Phosphatase And Tensin Homolog (PTEN), and Phosphatidylinositol-4,5-Bisphosphate 3-Kinase Catalytic Subunit Alpha (PIK3CA). Alterations in the mTOR pathway are highly investigated because drugs targeting the pathway (eg, everolimus) are efficacious in a subset of patients with advanced disease.[46,76] In patients without a family history, ~11% of PanNETs have germline mutations in the DNA damage repair pathway (eg, MutY DNA Glycosylase (MUTYH), Checkpoint Kinase 2 (CHEK2), and BRCA2 DNA Repair Associated (BRCA2)). Finally, a subset of PanNETs have somatic mutations affecting chromatin remodeling function (eg, ET Domain Containing 2, Histone Lysine Methyltransferase (SETD2) and AT-Rich Interaction Domain 1A (ARID1A)), which drives global transcriptional dysregulation. Highlighting the promising utility of these alterations as prognostic markers, Roy and colleagues[69] demonstrated that the loss of H3K36me3 protein expression (a surrogate for SETD2 mutation), the loss of ARID1A protein expression, and the presence of CDKN2A deletions are associated with reduced disease-specific survival.

In addition to the presence of specific gene mutations or mutational signatures, other groups have identified specific patterns of chromosomal copy number variations (CNVs) that can identify subgroups of PanNETs.[53,70,77–80] For example, Scarpa and colleagues[53] identified 4 groups: recurrent pattern of whole chromosomal loss, limited copy number (CN) events (mostly only affecting chromosome 11), polyploidy, and aneuploidy. Although focusing on small (<3 cm) primary PanNETs, Pea and colleagues identified 3 subgroups that displayed differing clinical risk for developing liver metastases. These groups were characterized by recurrent chromosomal gains and CN loss of heterozygosity (LOH) (73% metastasis rate), limited CN alterations (42% metastasis rate), or only chromosome 11 loss (35% metastasis rate).[70] Subsequent studies have linked these CNV profiles to the presence of specific mutational patterns. For example, PanNETs that exhibit a highly recurrent signature of LOH and CN alterations are strongly associated with mutations in either MEN1, ATRX, or DAXX (ie, MAD + tumors).[77] Similarly, Hong and colleagues[78] classified a cohort of 211 PanNETs (84 insulinomas and 127 NF-PanNETs) into subgroups based on mutational and CNV patterns and demonstrated insulinomas are vastly different from NF-PanNETs on a genomic level. Insulinomas either presented with CNV alterations (amplifications and copy neutral but lacking deletions) or as CNV-neutral with recurrent mutations in the transcription factor, YY1. In contrast, NF-PanNETs with CNV alterations (amplification and deletion) displayed a decreased relapse-free survival (RFS), whereas additional acquisition of a mutation in ATRX or DAXX further decreased the RFS time within the first 2 years.

Finally, in addition to evaluating genetic alterations in cancer tissue specimens, other groups have developed methodology to detect these alterations in a so-called liquid biopsy. For example, Boons and colleagues[81] provided proof-of-concept data from a small PanNET cohort demonstrating the feasibility of detecting cancer-specific mutations and CNV alterations in cell-free DNA from patients with metastatic disease. Similarly, Zakka and colleagues[82] has recently provided initial data demonstrating the feasibility of performing next generation sequencing testing using patient-derived circulating tumor DNA. Likely capturing the overall tumor biology, an assay that measures neuroendocrine tumor gene expression in blood (ie, transcriptomic signatures) has been developed and tested across various neuroendocrine tumors, including PanNETs.[83,84] In addition to accurately diagnosing the presence of a neuroendocrine tumor, this assay is also associated with the identification of a PanNET recurrence.[85,86]

EPIGENETIC SIGNATURES

As outlined previously, PanNETs commonly express hormones physiologically produced by endocrine pancreatic islets cells, and include glucagon (α-cells), insulin (β-cells), pancreatic polypeptide (γ-cells), and somatostatin (δ-cells).[87,88] Functioning PanNETs have long been classified by their clinically symptomatic hormone production, for which different types show markedly different prognosis (eg, insulinoma and glucagonoma). Until recently, NF-PanNETs were considered a single entity biologically, as well as prognostically. Although immunohistochemical hormone expression is regularly observed in NF-PanNETs, it is not routinely determined due to unpredictable and often focal multihormonal staining patterns, thereby leading to uncertain prognostic significance.[89,90]

Recently, several efforts have been made to classify NF-PanNETs based on endocrine differentiation, using more intricate epigenetic or transcriptomic signatures. Interestingly, although large differences existed in study populations and methodology, multiple research groups identified similar epigenetic NF-PanNETs subtypes with similarities resembling α-cells or β-cells and which were enriched for specific structural alterations and mutational profiles. Importantly, as highlighted in Table 3, these epigenetic signature subgroups were useful for predicting RFS.[91,92]

A study by Sadanandam and colleagues was the first to show that a subgroup of less aggressive NF-PanNETs has similarities to insulinomas, based on mRNA and miRNA transcriptome profiles. Typically, these insulinoma-like NF-PanNETs lacked MEN1, ATRX, or DAXX mutations, which were seen more often in the 2 other subgroups (intermediate and metastases-like).[93] Chan and colleagues later compared MEN1, ATRX, or DAXX (ADM)-mutant and wild-type PanNETs based on transcriptomic and DNA-methylation profiles, and

found ADM-mutant PanNETs cluster tightly together and have a uniform gene expression profile similar to α-cells. In comparison, ADM-wild-type PanNETs showed higher expression for some β-cell genes (including the transcription factor, Pancreatic And Duodenal Homeobox 1 [PDX1]) but also exhibited greater heterogeneity in the gene expression.[91] Cejas and colleagues identified 3 PanNET subgroups based on H3K27-acetylation enhancer profiles. Differential enhancer acetylation and gene expression of Aristaless Related Homeobox (ARX) (normally expressed in α, γ, and ε-cells but not in β-cells) and PDX1 (normally expressed in β, γ, δ, and ε-cells but not in α-cells) in 2 out of 3 PanNET signatures prompted an immunohistochemical evaluation of ARX/PDX1 protein expression in a larger series of sporadic and Menin 1 (MEN1)-associated NF-PanNETs.[87,88,92] Interestingly, in a multiple logistic regression analysis of 83 NF-PanNETs, only the presence of ALT or lack of PDX1 expression independently correlated with relapse. PDX1 expressing PanNETs rarely relapsed and were associated with a lack of ALT.[92]

Because of these interesting findings, a recent large multi-institutional study for the validation of novel PanNET biomarkers performed ARX/PDX1 immunohistochemistry on 561 primary sporadic NF-PanNETs. Surprisingly, although ARX and PDX1 were expressed in 72% and 43% of NF-PanNETs respectively, no value was found in univariate and multivariate survival analyses to predict RFS.[41] Only the strong association of ARX expression or the lack of PDX1 expression with ATRX/DAXX protein loss and the presence of ALT was confirmed, and a possible role of these markers was suggested to predict the origin of neuroendocrine tumors of unknown primary.[41]

These discrepant results may be explained by differences in study characteristics (only sporadic tumors vs partially MEN1-associated). Moreover, recent studies suggest that ARX and PDX1 immunohistochemistry might not be optimal surrogate markers of epigenetic signatures. Di Domenico and colleagues[94] performed an elegant phylo-epigenetic analysis of 125 PanNETs (both functional and nonfunctional), using normal α-cells and β-cells as root nodes. The PanNETs were divided into 3 arbitrary groups based on a phylo-epigenetic tree. The group nearest to β-cells consisted almost entirely of insulinomas. PDX1 expression was present in all insulinomas but, in contrast to previous studies, in none of the NF-PanNETs; however, different antibodies were used across the studies.[41,92,94–96] The group closest to α-cells (mostly NF-PanNETs) was characterized by MEN1 mutations, limited CN events,

Table 3
Pancreatic neuroendocrine tumor classification based on genetic and epigenetic signatures

	Global Summary					
	NF-PanNET 1	**NF-PanNET 2**	**NF-PanNET 3**	**Insulinoma 1**	**Insulinoma 2**	**Insulinoma 3[a]**
Epigenetic similarities	α-cell-like	α-cell-like>β-cell-like	β-cell-like/other	β-cell-like	β-cell-like	α-cell-like>β-cell-like
Epigenetic signature	Well-differentiated	Dedifferentiated	Unknown	Well-differentiated	Well-differentiated	Dedifferentiated?
MEN1	++	+++	+/−	−	−	U
ATRX/DAXX	+	+++	−	−	−	++
YY1	−	−	−	+++	−	U
mTOR	+	+++	+	−	−	U
Copy number profiles	Copy number neutral	Copy number amplifications/deletions	Copy number neutral	Copy number neutral	Recurrent amplifications	U
Predominant Grade	G1	G2	G1	G1	G1	G2
Mean size	3 cm	4 cm	3 cm	< 2 cm	< 2 cm	> 3 cm
Prognosis	Favorable	Poor	Favorable	Favorable	Favorable	Poor
Approximate overlap of PanNET epigenetic and copy number subtypes						
Sadanandam et al,[93] 2015	MLP/Intermediate-type		Insulinoma-like			
Chan et al,[91] 2018	ADM-mutant	ADM-mutant	ADM-wild-type			ADM-mutant
Di Domenico et al,[94] 2020	α-tumors	Intermediate-tumors	β-tumors			Intermediate-tumors
Boons et al,[97] 2020	Subtype A		Subtype B			
Lakis et al,[98] 2021	T3	T2	T1			
Cejas et al,[92] 2019	PDX-negative		PDX1-positive	ARX-negative		
Hackeng et al,[96] 2020	−		ARX-negative			ARX-positive
Hong et al,[78] 2020	NF-Neutral	NF-Amp/Del	NF-Neutral	Ins-Neu	Ins-Amp	−

Summary of recent insights in surgically resected sporadic PanNET subtypes, main subgroups based on Hong et al.[78] and other studies are matched based on clinical characteristics, copy number profiling, recurrent mutations, and differentiation.

Abbreviations: ADM, *ATRX, DAXX,* or *MEN1* mutant; G, World Health Organization grade; MLP, metastases-like primary; NF-PanNET, non-functional pancreatic neuroendocrine tumor; u, unknown.

[a] Possibly the same as NF-PanNET-2 with acquired symptomatic insulin production.

and no *ATRX* or *DAXX* mutations. Tumors in between, called the intermediate group, showed varying degrees of similarity to both α-cells and β-cells. The intermediate group was characterized by recurrent *MEN1*, *ATRX*, and *DAXX* mutations and frequent CN aberrations. Although most of both the α-like and intermediate PanNETs displayed immunohistochemical ARX expression, α-like PanNETs had significantly longer DFS compared with the "intermediate" PanNETs. Interestingly, the α-like and intermediate PanNETs seem to overlap with the NF-neutral and NF-Del/Amp groups described by Hong and colleagues,[78] respectively. Unfortunately, ARX immunohistochemistry would fail to discriminate between "α-like/NF-neutral" and "intermediate/NF-Del/Amp" PanNETs.

Based on these and several other studies,[95,97,98] it seems that ARX expression or a lack of PDX1 expression associates with a genetic pathway of tumorigenesis, rather than a specific epigenetic signature. Two types of ARX-positive NF-PanNETs can be encountered: the first group has strong α-cell characteristics, limited CNVs, and recurrent *MEN1* mutations and the second group has less pronounced α-cell characteristics, significant CN alterations, and in addition to *MEN1* mutations, recurrent *ATRX* or *DAXX* mutations leading to the activation of ALT. It seems plausible that PanNETs with strong α-cell characteristics can progress to the intermediate group as a result of additional chromosomal instability and mutations causing α-cell dedifferentiation. However, it is unclear if β-cell tumors (or other endocrine cell tumors) that acquire *MEN1* or *ATRX/DAXX* mutations might also contribute to this intermediate dedifferentiated group. In this regard, reported α-cell transdifferentiation in murine *MEN1*-mutant β-cell tumors is of interest.[99]

Few studies have focused on the epigenetic signatures of functional tumors. In fact, only insulinomas have sufficiently been studied. As expected, most insulinomas have strong epigenetic similarities to β-cells (PDX1-positive/ARX-negative).[93,94,96] However, some rare insulinomas do express ARX and are further characterized by large tumor size (3.5–9 cm) and metastatic behavior.[96] Interestingly, these ARX-positive insulinomas were most often ALT-positive, again confirming ARX-expression as marker of a genetic pathway of tumorigenesis. However, the origin of these large metastatic ARX-positive insulinomas may be different from the typical small insulinomas commonly detected. Typical insulinomas become symptomatic very early when they are small in size (<2 cm). In contrast, ARX-positive insulinomas are all much larger and, therefore, most likely existed

as NF-PanNETs for a time before becoming clinically functional.[96] However, it is unknown if the insulin production was already present in these NF-PanNETs at asymptomatic levels. Moreover, the initiating molecular events leading to ARX-positive insulinomas are unclear. Potential hypotheses include a nonfunctional β-cell tumor that acquired α-cell characteristics (possibly after *ATRX/DAXX* mutations and presence of ALT) or a nonfunctional α-cell/intermediate tumor that acquired β-cell characteristics (ie, insulin production).

SUMMARY AND PERSPECTIVE

As illustrated, the wide pathologic heterogeneity among PanNETs results in different clinical behaviors and treatment responses. The currently used WHO grading classification and TNM staging have limitations as prognostic parameters because preoperative grading of PanNETs on cytologic specimens is unreliable[95] and the prognostic value of tumor size remains controversial. Therefore, novel prognostic biomarkers, that can also be assessed preoperatively, are needed to improve the stratification and treatment of patients with PanNETs.

Numerous retrospective studies have independently validated ALT and/or ATRX/DAXX loss as prognostic biomarkers associated with adverse prognostic features, most notably the presence of metastatic disease and reduced RFS.[41,55–57,64] Importantly, a recent study demonstrated that ALT and/or ATRX/DAXX loss are independent prognostic biomarkers in small (<2 cm) PanNETs. Because ALT and ATRX/DAXX loss can be reliably assessed in cytologic specimens,[95,100] these are potential promising preoperative biomarkers that may be able to stratify patients for active surveillance versus surgical resection. Prospective studies are now urgently needed to validate ALT and ATRX/DAXX loss for this purpose.

Moreover, other less frequent mutations in PanNETs may have prognostic value. In this regard, loss of H3K36me3 expression, loss of ARID1A protein expression, and the presence of *CDKN2A* deletions have been associated with reduced DFS.[69] In addition, chromosomal CNV patterns have successfully been used in identifying subgroups of PanNETs that are associated with different risks of developing metastatic disease and the presence of specific mutational patterns.

Recent transcriptomic and epigenetic studies focusing on endocrine differentiation to classify NF-PanNETs have shed new light on PanNET pathologic condition. Despite differences between studies, basically 3 different epigenetic NF-PanNET subtypes can be dissected with similarities to α-cells or β-cells, specific structural alterations, mutational profiles, and significant prognostic differences (see Table 3). The first subgroup displays strong α-cell characteristics, recurrent *MEN1* mutations, limited CNVs, and a relatively good prognosis. The second subgroup displays less pronounced α-cell characteristics, *MEN1* mutations, additional *ATRX* or *DAXX* mutations leading to the activation of ALT, significant CNVs, and a relatively poor prognosis. The third subgroup displays strong β-cell characteristics, limited CNVs, and a relatively good prognosis. It seems plausible that PanNETs with strong α-cell characteristics may progress into the intermediate group due to accumulation of additional chromosomal instability and mutations causing α-cell dedifferentiation. In contrast, whether PanNETs with strong β-cell characteristics, that ultimately acquire *MEN1* or *ATRX/DAXX* mutations, can similarly progress to this intermediate dedifferentiated group remains unclear.[91,92]

Future studies evaluating these epigenetic signatures need to address several challenges before they can be routinely incorporated into clinical practice. First, for prognostic studies, functional PanNETs (particularly insulinomas) and NF-PanNETs should always be separately analyzed when evaluating survival outcomes because their clinical presentations and prognoses are dramatically different.[78] Second, most described molecular subgroups are based on unsupervised clustering methods. For clinical applicability, a specific set of genes/CpG sites or inexpensive surrogate markers should be selected and a predictive model built to classify new cases. Finally, the added value of these epigenetic signatures need to be directly compared in multivariate survival analyses with established markers of PanNET behavior, such as WHO grade, ALT or copy-number variations, and/or novel markers (eg, H&E deep-learning based prediction models[101]), especially because these are likely to be highly associated with each other.

To conclude, genetic and recent epigenetic insights have greatly changed the way we look at PanNETs but many questions remain unanswered. Future comprehensive prospective studies combining genetic and epigenetic data in cohorts of primary PanNETs with detailed clinical follow-up data are needed to fully elucidate the relationship between epigenetic profiles, mutational signatures, and CNV profiles. This may lead to more definitive and clinically useful PanNET subtyping that will optimize and personalize patient treatments.

CLINICS CARE POINTS

- ALT and ATRX/DAXX protein loss as poor prognostic biomarkers in primary non-syndromic/non-functional PanNETs without distant metastases at surgical resection.
- In small (<2 cm) PanNETs, ALT and ATRX/DAXX protein loss are independent prognostic biomarkers for decreased recurrence-free survival.

DISCLOSURE

The authors do not have any commercial or financial conflicts of interest. This study is supported by the Dutch Cancer Society (KWF grant 12978 to L.A.A. Brosens) and by the American Cancer Society (Boston University-Boston Medical Center Pilot and Feasibility Program to C.M. Heaphy).

REFERENCES

1. Ma Z-Y, Gong Y-F, Zhuang H-K, et al. Pancreatic neuroendocrine tumors: a review of serum biomarkers, staging, and management. World J Gastroenterol 2020;26:2305–22.
2. Fang JM, Shi J. A clinicopathologic and molecular update of pancreatic neuroendocrine neoplasms with a focus on the new world health organization classification. Arch Pathol Lab Med 2019;143:1317–26.
3. Yadav S, Sharma P, Zakalik D. Comparison of demographics, tumor characteristics, and survival between pancreatic adenocarcinomas and pancreatic neuroendocrine tumors: a population-based study. Am J Clin Oncol 2016;41:1.
4. Halfdanarson TR, Rabe KG, Rubin J, et al. Pancreatic neuroendocrine tumors (PNETs): incidence, prognosis and recent trend toward improved survival. Ann Oncol 2008;19:1727–33.
5. Cloyd JM, Poultsides GA. Non-functional neuroendocrine tumors of the pancreas: advances in diagnosis and management. World J Gastroenterol 2015;21:9512–25.
6. Scott AT, Howe JR. Evaluation and management of neuroendocrine tumors of the pancreas. Surg Clin North Am 2019;99:793–814.
7. Lee DW, Kim MK, Kim HG. Diagnosis of pancreatic neuroendocrine tumors. Clin Endosc 2017;50:537–45.
8. Jensen RT, Cadiot G, Brandi ML, et al. Barcelona Consensus Conference p. ENETS Consensus Guidelines for the management of patients with digestive neuroendocrine neoplasms: functional

pancreatic endocrine tumor syndromes. Neuroen-docrinology 2012;95:98–119.

9. Okabayashi T, Shima Y, Sumiyoshi T, et al. Diagnosis and management of insulinoma. World J Gastroenterol 2013;19:829–37.

10. Anlauf M, Garbrecht N, Bauersfeld J, et al. Hereditary neuroendocrine tumors of the gastroenteropancreatic system. *Virchows Arch*, 541, 2007, S29-38.

11. Jensen RT, Berna MJ, Bingham DB, et al. Inherited pancreatic endocrine tumor syndromes: advances in molecular pathogenesis, diagnosis, management, and controversies. Cancer 2008;113:1807–43.

12. Geurts JL. Inherited syndromes involving pancreatic neuroendocrine tumors. J Gastrointest Oncol 2020;11:559–66.

13. Pea A, Hruban RH, Wood LD. Genetics of pancreatic neuroendocrine tumors: implications for the clinic. Expert Rev Gastroenterol Hepatol 2015;9:1407–19.

14. Thakker RV, Newey PJ, Walls GV, et al. Clinical practice guidelines for multiple endocrine neoplasia type 1 (MEN1). J Clin Endocrinol Metab 2012;97:2990–3011.

15. Kamilaris CDC, Stratakis CA. Multiple endocrine neoplasia type 1 (MEN1): an update and the significance of early genetic and clinical diagnosis. Front Endocrinol 2019;10:339.

16. Tamura K, Nishimori I, Ito T, et al. Diagnosis and management of pancreatic neuroendocrine tumor in von Hippel-Lindau disease. World J Gastroenterol 2010;16:4515–8.

17. Ito T, Igarashi H, Jensen RT. Pancreatic neuroendocrine tumors: clinical features, diagnosis and medical treatment: advances. Best Pract Res Clin Gastroenterol 2012;26:737–53.

18. Iacovazzo D, Flanagan SE, Walker E, et al. MAFA missense mutation causes familial insulinomatosis and diabetes mellitus. Proc Natl Acad Sci U S A 2018;115:1027–32.

19. Sipos B, Sperveslage J, Anlauf M, et al. Glucagon cell hyperplasia and neoplasia with and without glucagon receptor mutations. J Clin Endocrinol Metab 2015;100:E783–8.

20. Bocchini M, Nicolini F, Severi S, et al. Biomarkers for pancreatic neuroendocrine neoplasms (PanNENs) management-an updated review. Front Oncol 2020;10:831.

21. Lee L, Ito T, Jensen RT. Prognostic and predictive factors on overall survival and surgical outcomes in pancreatic neuroendocrine tumors: recent advances and controversies. Expert Rev Anticancer Ther 2019;19:1029–50.

22. Pavel M, Oberg K, Falconi M, et al. Gastroenteropancreatic neuroendocrine neoplasms: ESMO Clinical Practice Guidelines for diagnosis, treatment and follow-up. Ann Oncol 2020;31:844–60.

23. Nagtegaal ID, Odze RD, Klimstra D, et al. The 2019 WHO classification of tumours of the digestive system. Histopathology 2020;76:182–8.

24. Assarzadegan N, Montgomery E. What is new in the 2019 World Health Organization (WHO) classification of tumors of the digestive system: review of selected updates on neuroendocrine neoplasms, appendiceal tumors, and molecular testing. Arch Pathol Lab Med 2021;145:664–77.

25. Yang M, Zeng L, Ke NW, et al. World Health Organization grading classification for pancreatic neuroendocrine neoplasms: a comprehensive analysis from a large Chinese institution. BMC Cancer 2020;20:906.

26. Pezzilli R, Partelli S, Cannizzaro R, et al. Ki-67 prognostic and therapeutic decision driven marker for pancreatic neuroendocrine neoplasms (PNENs): A systematic review. Adv Med Sci 2016;61:147–53.

27. Nadler A, Cukier M, Rowsell C, et al. Ki-67 is a reliable pathological grading marker for neuroendocrine tumors. Virchows Arch 2013;462:501–5.

28. Philips P, Kooby DA, Maithel S, et al. Grading using Ki-67 index and mitotic rate increases the prognostic accuracy of pancreatic neuroendocrine tumors. Pancreas 2018;47:326–31.

29. McCall CM, Shi C, Cornish TC, et al. Grading of well-differentiated pancreatic neuroendocrine tumors is improved by the inclusion of both Ki67 proliferative index and mitotic rate. Am J Surg Pathol 2013;37:1671–7.

30. Brunner P, Jorg AC, Glatz K, et al. The prognostic and predictive value of sstr2-immunohistochemistry and sstr2-targeted imaging in neuroendocrine tumors. Eur J Nucl Med Mol Imaging 2017;44:468–75.

31. Okuwaki K, Kida M, Mikami T, et al. Clinicopathologic characteristics of pancreatic neuroendocrine tumors and relation of somatostatin receptor type 2A to outcomes. Cancer 2013;119:4094–102.

32. Gao S, Pu N, Liu L, et al. The latest exploration of staging and prognostic classification for pancreatic neuroendocrine tumors: a large population based study. J Cancer 2018;9:1698–706.

33. Hamilton NA, Liu TC, Cavatiao A, et al. Ki-67 predicts disease recurrence and poor prognosis in pancreatic neuroendocrine neoplasms. Surgery 2012;152:107–13.

34. Bettini R, Partelli S, Boninsegna L, et.al. Tumor size correlates with malignancy in nonfunctioning pancreatic endocrine tumor. Surgery 2011;150:75–82.

35. Gao Y, Gao H, Wang G, et al. A meta-analysis of Prognostic factor of Pancreatic neuroendocrine neoplasms. Sci Rep 2018;8:7271.

36. Assi HA, Mukherjee S, Kunz PL, et al. Surgery versus surveillance for well-differentiated, nonfunctional pancreatic neuroendocrine tumors: an 11-

year analysis of the national cancer database. Oncologist 2020;25:e276–83.

37. Halfdanarson TR, Strosberg JR, Tang L, et al. The North American neuroendocrine tumor society consensus guidelines for surveillance and medical management of pancreatic neuroendocrine tumors. Pancreas 2020;49:863–81.

38. Falconi M, Eriksson B, Kaltsas G, et al. ENETS consensus guidelines update for the management of patients with functional pancreatic neuroendocrine tumors and non-functional pancreatic neuroendocrine tumors. Neuroendocrinology 2016;103: 153–71.

39. Sadot E, Reidy-Lagunes DL, Tang LH, et al. Observation versus resection for small asymptomatic pancreatic neuroendocrine tumors: a matched case-control study. Ann Surg Oncol 2016;23: 1361–70.

40. Haynes AB, Deshpande V, Ingkakul T, et al. Implications of incidentally discovered, nonfunctioning pancreatic endocrine tumors: short-term and long-term patient outcomes. Arch Surg 2011;146: 534–8.

41. Hackeng WM, Brosens LAA, Kim JY, et al. Nonfunctional pancreatic neuroendocrine tumours: ATRX/DAXX and alternative lengthening of telomeres (ALT) are prognostically independent from ARX/PDX1 expression and tumour size. Gut 2022; 71:961–73.

42. Partelli S, Ramage JK, Massironi S, et al. Management of asymptomatic sporadic nonfunctioning pancreatic neuroendocrine neoplasms (ASPEN) </=2 cm: study protocol for a prospective observational study. Front Med (Lausanne) 2020;7:598438.

43. Mayo SC, de Jong MC, Pulitano C, et al. Surgical management of hepatic neuroendocrine tumor metastasis: results from an international multi-institutional analysis. Ann Surg Oncol 2010;17: 3129–36.

44. Scott AT, Breheny PJ, Keck KJ, et al. Effective cytoreduction can be achieved in patients with numerous neuroendocrine tumor liver metastases (NETLMs). Surgery 2019;165:166–75.

45. Caplin ME, Pavel M, Cwikla JB, et al. Lanreotide in metastatic enteropancreatic neuroendocrine tumors. N Engl J Med 2014;371:224–33.

46. Yao JC, Shah MH, Ito T, et al. Rad001 in Advanced Neuroendocrine Tumors TTSG. Everolimus for advanced pancreatic neuroendocrine tumors. N Engl J Med 2011;364:514–23.

47. Faivre S, Niccoli P, Castellano D, et al. Sunitinib in pancreatic neuroendocrine tumors: updated progression-free survival and final overall survival from a phase III randomized study. Ann Oncol 2017;28:339–43.

48. Strosberg JR, Caplin ME, Kunz PL, et al, group obotN-s. Final overall survival in the phase 3 NETTER-1 study of lutetium-177-DOTATATE in patients with midgut neuroendocrine tumors. J Clin Oncol 2021;39:4112.

49. de Mestier L, Walter T, Evrard C, et al. Temozolomide Alone or Combined with Capecitabine for the Treatment of Advanced Pancreatic Neuroendocrine Tumor. Neuroendocrinology 2020;110: 83–91.

50. Al-Toubah T, Morse B, Pelle E, et al. Efficacy of FOLFOX in Patients with Aggressive Pancreatic Neuroendocrine Tumors After Prior Capecitabine/Temozolomide. Oncologist 2021;26:115–9.

51. Thomas KEH, Voros BA, Boudreaux JP, et al. Current Treatment Options in Gastroenteropancreatic Neuroendocrine Carcinoma. Oncologist 2019;24: 1076–88.

52. Jiao Y, Shi C, Edil BH, et al. DAXX/ATRX, MEN1, and mTOR pathway genes are frequently altered in pancreatic neuroendocrine tumors. Science 2011;331:1199–203.

53. Scarpa A, Chang DK, Nones K, et al. Whole-genome landscape of pancreatic neuroendocrine tumours. Nature 2017;543:65–71.

54. Li JWY, Hua X, Reidy-Lagunes D, et al. MENIN loss as a tissue-specific driver of tumorigenesis. Mol Cell Endocrinol 2018;469:98–106.

55. Singhi AD, Liu TC, Roncaioli JL, et al. Alternative lengthening of telomeres and loss of DAXX/ATRX expression predicts metastatic disease and poor survival in patients with pancreatic neuroendocrine tumors. Clin Cancer Res 2017;23:600–9.

56. Kim JY, Brosnan-Cashman JA, An S, et al. Alternative lengthening of telomeres in primary pancreatic neuroendocrine tumors is associated with aggressive clinical behavior and poor survival. Clin Cancer Res 2017;23:1598–606.

57. Marinoni I, Kurrer AS, Vassella E, et al. Loss of DAXX and ATRX are associated with chromosome instability and reduced survival of patients with pancreatic neuroendocrine tumors. Gastroenterology 2014;146:453–460 e455.

58. Heaphy CM, de Wilde RF, Jiao Y, et al. Altered telomeres in tumors with ATRX and DAXX mutations. Science 2011;333:425.

59. Lovejoy CA, Li W, Reisenweber S, et al. Loss of ATRX, genome instability, and an altered DNA damage response are hallmarks of the alternative lengthening of telomeres pathway. PLoS Genet 2012;8:e1002772.

60. Lewis PW, Elsaesser SJ, Noh KM, et al. Daxx is an H3.3-specific histone chaperone and cooperates with ATRX in replication-independent chromatin assembly at telomeres. Proc Natl Acad Sci U S A 2010;107:14075–80.

61. Dilley RL, Greenberg RA. ALTernative telomere maintenance and cancer. Trends Cancer 2015;1: 145–56.

62. de Wilde RF, Heaphy CM, Maitra A, et al. Loss of ATRX or DAXX expression and concomitant acquisition of the alternative lengthening of telomeres phenotype are late, events in a small subset of MEN-1 syndrome pancreatic neuroendocrine tumors. Mod Pathol 2012;25:1033–9.

63. Hackeng WM, Brosens LA, Poruk KE, et al. Aberrant Menin expression is an early event in pancreatic neuroendocrine tumorigenesis. Hum Pathol 2016;56:93–100.

64. Pipinikas CP, Dibra H, Karpathakis A, et al. Epigenetic dysregulation and poorer prognosis in DAXX-deficient pancreatic neuroendocrine tumours. Endocr Relat Cancer 2015;22:L13–8.

65. Cives M, Partelli S, Palmirotta R, et al. DAXX mutations as potential genomic markers of malignant evolution in small nonfunctioning pancreatic neuroendocrine tumors. Sci Rep 2019;9:18614.

66. Ziv E, Rice SL, Filtes J, et al. DAXX mutation status of embolization-treated neuroendocrine tumors predicts shorter time to hepatic progression. J Vasc Interv Radiol 2018;29:1519–26.

67. Chou A, Itchins M, de Reuver PR, et al. ATRX loss is an independent predictor of poor survival in pancreatic neuroendocrine tumors. Hum Pathol 2018;82:249–57.

68. Park JK, Paik WH, Lee K, et al. DAXX/ATRX and MEN1 genes are strong prognostic markers in pancreatic neuroendocrine tumors. Oncotarget 2017;8:49796–806.

69. Roy S, LaFramboise WA, Liu TC, et al. Loss of chromatin-remodeling proteins and/or CDKN2A associates with metastasis of pancreatic neuroendocrine tumors and reduced patient survival times. Gastroenterology 2018;154:2060–2063 e2068.

70. Pea A, Yu J, Marchionni L, et al. Genetic analysis of small well-differentiated pancreatic neuroendocrine tumors identifies subgroups with differing risks of liver metastases. Ann Surg 2020;271:566–73.

71. Luchini C, Lawlor RT, Bersani S, et al. Alternative lengthening of telomeres (ALT) in pancreatic neuroendocrine tumors: ready for prime-time in clinical practice? Curr Oncol Rep 2021;23:106.

72. Marinoni I. Prognostic value of DAXX/ATRX loss of expression and ALT activation in PanNETs: is it time for clinical implementation? Gut 2022;71:847–8.

73. Raj N, Shah R, Stadler Z, et al. Real-time genomic characterization of metastatic pancreatic neuroendocrine tumors has prognostic implications and identifies potential germline actionability. JCO Precis Oncol 2018;2018. https://doi.org/10.1200/PO.17.00267.

74. van Riet J, van de Werken HJG, Cuppen E, et al. The genomic landscape of 85 advanced neuroendocrine neoplasms reveals subtype-heterogeneity and potential therapeutic targets. Nat Commun 2021;12:4612.

75. Wong HL, Yang KC, Shen Y, et al. Molecular characterization of metastatic pancreatic neuroendocrine tumors (PNETs) using whole-genome and transcriptome sequencing. Cold Spring Harb Mol Case Stud 2018;4:a002329.

76. Yao JC, Phan AT, Jehl V, et al. Everolimus in advanced pancreatic neuroendocrine tumors: the clinical experience. Cancer Res 2013;73:1449–53.

77. Quevedo R, Spreafico A, Bruce J, et al. Centromeric cohesion failure invokes a conserved choreography of chromosomal mis-segregations in pancreatic neuroendocrine tumor. Genome Med 2020;12:38.

78. Hong X, Qiao S, Li F, et al. Whole-genome sequencing reveals distinct genetic bases for insulinomas and non-functional pancreatic neuroendocrine tumours: leading to a new classification system. Gut 2020;69:877–87.

79. Yao J, Garg A, Chen D, et al. Genomic profiling of NETs: a comprehensive analysis of the RADIANT trials. Endocr Relat Cancer 2019;26:391–403.

80. Lawrence B, Blenkiron C, Parker K, et al. Recurrent loss of heterozygosity correlates with clinical outcome in pancreatic neuroendocrine cancer. NPJ Genom Med 2018;3:18.

81. Boons G, Vandamme T, Peeters M, et al. Cell-free DNA from metastatic pancreatic neuroendocrine tumor patients contains tumor-specific mutations and copy number variations. Front Oncol 2018;8:467.

82. Zakka K, Nagy R, Drusbosky L, et al. Blood-based next-generation sequencing analysis of neuroendocrine neoplasms. Oncotarget 2020;11:1749–57.

83. Modlin IM, Kidd M, Malczewska A, et al. The NETest: the clinical utility of multigene blood analysis in the diagnosis and management of neuroendocrine tumors. Endocrinol Metab Clin North Am 2018;47:485–504.

84. Malczewska A, Kos-Kudla B, Kidd M, et al. The clinical applications of a multigene liquid biopsy (NETest) In neuroendocrine tumors. Adv Med Sci 2020;65:18–29.

85. Genc CG, Jilesen APJ, Nieveen van Dijkum EJM, et al. Measurement of circulating transcript levels (NETest) to detect disease recurrence and improve follow-up after curative surgical resection of well-differentiated pancreatic neuroendocrine tumors. J Surg Oncol 2018;118:37–48.

86. Oberg K, Califano A, Strosberg JR, et al. A meta-analysis of the accuracy of a neuroendocrine tumor mRNA genomic biomarker (NETest) in blood. Ann Oncol 2020;31:202–12.

87. Muraro MJ, Dharmadhikari G, Grun D, et al. A single-cell transcriptome atlas of the human pancreas. Cell Syst 2016;3:385–394 e383.

88. Baron M, Veres A, Wolock SL, et al. A single-cell transcriptomic map of the human and mouse pancreas reveals inter- and intra-cell population structure. Cell Syst 2016;3:346–360 e344.

89. Hochwald SN, Zee S, Conlon KC, et al. Prognostic factors in pancreatic endocrine neoplasms: an analysis of 136 cases with a proposal for low-grade and intermediate-grade groups. J Clin Oncol 2002;20:2633–42.

90. Kapran Y, Bauersfeld J, Anlauf M, et al. Multihormonality and entrapment of islets in pancreatic endocrine tumors. Virchows Arch 2006;448:394–8.

91. Chan CS, Laddha SV, Lewis PW, et al. ATRX, DAXX or MEN1 mutant pancreatic neuroendocrine tumors are a distinct alpha-cell signature subgroup. Nat Commun 2018;9:4158.

92. Cejas P, Drier Y, Dreijerink KMA, et al. Enhancer signatures stratify and predict outcomes of non-functional pancreatic neuroendocrine tumors. Nat Med 2019;25:1260–5.

93. Sadanandam A, Wullschleger S, Lyssiotis CA, et al. A cross-species analysis in pancreatic neuroendocrine tumors reveals molecular subtypes with distinctive clinical, metastatic, developmental, and metabolic characteristics. Cancer Discov 2015;5: 1296–313.

94. Di Domenico A, Pipinikas CP, Maire RS, et al. Epigenetic landscape of pancreatic neuroendocrine tumours reveals distinct cells of origin and means of tumour progression. Commun Biol 2020;3:740.

95. Hackeng WM, Morsink FHM, Moons LMG, et al. Assessment of ARX expression, a novel biomarker for metastatic risk in pancreatic neuroendocrine tumors, in endoscopic ultrasound fine-needle aspiration. Diagn Cytopathol 2020;48:308–15.

96. Hackeng WM, Schelhaas W, Morsink FHM, et al. Alternative lengthening of telomeres and differential expression of endocrine transcription factors distinguish metastatic and non-metastatic insulinomas. Endocr Pathol 2020;31:108–18.

97. Boons G, Vandamme T, Ibrahim J, et al. PDX1 DNA methylation distinguishes two subtypes of pancreatic neuroendocrine neoplasms with a different prognosis. Cancers (Basel) 2020;12:1461.

98. Lakis V, Lawlor RT, Newell F, et al. DNA methylation patterns identify subgroups of pancreatic neuroendocrine tumors with clinical association. Commun Biol 2021;4:155.

99. Li F, Su Y, Cheng Y, et al. Conditional deletion of Men1 in the pancreatic beta-cell leads to glucagon-expressing tumor development. Endocrinology 2015;156:48–57.

100. VandenBussche CJ, Allison DB, Graham MK, et al. Alternative lengthening of telomeres and ATRX/DAXX loss can be reliably detected in FNAs of pancreatic neuroendocrine tumors. Cancer Cytopathol 2017;125:544–51.

101. Klimov S, Xue Y, Gertych A, et al. Predicting metastasis risk in pancreatic neuroendocrine tumors using deep learning image analysis. Front Oncol 2020;10:593211.

Mixed Neuroendocrine-Non-Neuroendocrine Neoplasms of the Pancreas

Vassilena Tsvetkova, MD, PhD, Claudio Luchini, MD, PhD*

KEYWORDS

- Mixed pancreatic tumors • MiNEN • MANEC • Neuroendocrine

Key points

- Pancreatic mixed neuroendocrine-non-neuroendocrine neoplasms (MiNENs) are mixed neoplasms, with the neuroendocrine component always represented.
- The diagnosis of pancreatic MiNEN should be based on morphology and immunohistochemistry.
- Each component should be specifically described in the final pathology report.
- The prognosis of this entity is very heterogeneous and depends on the different tumor components.

ABSTRACT

Pancreatic mixed neuroendocrine-non-neuroendocrine neoplasms (MiNENs) are rare neoplasms, composed of at least two components. The neuroendocrine part is always present. Histology is the most important tool for the diagnosis, but in the case of MiNEN, it is also important for the use of immunohistochemistry, which should include neuroendocrine but also ductal and acinar markers. Each component should be specifically described in the final pathology report, including the percentage on the entire tumor mass. The prognosis of MiNEN is very heterogeneous and depends on the different tumor components.

INTRODUCTION

Pancreatic mixed neuroendocrine-non-neuroendocrine neoplasms (MiNENs) are a heterogeneous group of mixed tumors composed of morphologically recognizable endocrine and non-endocrine components, each of which representing at least 30% of the tumor volume.[1] The specific etiology of this heterogeneous entity remains unknown. The non-endocrine component is represented by pancreatic ductal adenocarcinoma or by acinar cell carcinoma, whereas the endocrine component, which is always present, is mainly represented by neuroendocrine carcinoma (NEC), although few cases of neuroendocrine tumors (NETs) in this setting have been reported as well.

Mixed ductal-NEC is a very rare entity and represents up to 1% of all ductal adenocarcinoma; patients with this kind of neoplasm have an average age at the diagnosis that falls into the seventh decade.[2] There is no significant difference in the incidence of this entity between man and women. Mixed acinar cell-NECs are also considered rare neoplasms, and they represent up to 15% of all pancreatic acinar cell carcinomas.[3,4] Also, for this MiNEN subtype, there is not a gender-based prevalence, and the average age at diagnosis falls between the sixth and the seventh decade.[1]

During the last years, various nomenclatures have been adopted. Initially, to describe mixed neoplasms composed of adenocarcinoma and endocrine components, Lewin and colleagues[5] in 1987 proposed a classification of mixed neoplasms into three subcategories: (i) collision tumors, (ii) combined tumors, and (iii) amphicrine tumors. This classification was not worldwide adopted, and only in 2000s, the first attempt to

Department of Diagnostics and Public Health, Section of Pathology, University and Hospital Trust of Verona, Piazzale Scuro, 10, Verona 37134, Italy
* Corresponding author.
E-mail address: claudio.luchini@univr.it

Surgical Pathology 15 (2022) 555–563
https://doi.org/10.1016/j.path.2022.05.008
1875-9181/22/© 2022 Elsevier Inc. All rights reserved.

surgpath.theclinics.com

Table 1
Current classification and possible composition of pancreatic mixed neuroendocrine-non-neuroendocrine neoplasms

Ductal Adenocarcinoma	NEC • Small cell NEC • Large cell NEC
Acinar cell carcinoma	NEC • Small cell NEC • Large cell NEC
Ductal adenocarcinoma–acinar cell carcinoma	NEC • Small cell NEC • Large cell NEC
Ductal adenocarcinoma	NET • G1 • G2 • G3
Acinar cell carcinoma	NET • G1 • G2 • G3

As indicated (right column), the neuroendocrine component is a constant presence.

Abbreviations: NEC, neuroendocrine carcinoma; NET, neuroendocrine tumor.

standardize the terminology was made by Capella and colleagues.[6] They called the mixed neoplasms as "Mixed exocrine-endocrine tumors," and this terminology was also acknowledged by the World Health Organization (WHO) classification.[7] With this definition, for the first time, the 30% of cutoff for each component was introduced as an essential diagnostic criterion for such mixed neoplasms. Although it may appear as an arbitrary threshold, this criterion is still currently applied.

In 2010, the WHO classification changed the nomenclature to "Mixed AdenoNeuroEndocrine Carcinoma (MANEC)."[8] This change was approved because most of mixed neoplasms were composed of adenocarcinoma and NEC. However, there was a growing evidence that MANEC category was much more heterogeneous, thus in 2019, the WHO classification this term was replaced by "MiNEN," also acknowledging that the neuroendocrine component could be represented even by low-grade NETs.[9] The latest classification of MiNEN is represented in **Table 1**.

Patients with MiNEN do not present specific symptoms, which are usually the result of a mass effect or are caused by the presence of distant metastases. Most commonly observed symptoms include poorly localized pain, weight loss, and gastrointestinal disturbances.

GROSS FEATURES

Macroscopically, MiNENs that include a ductal adenocarcinoma as the non-endocrine component are usually large and solid tumors, with undefined margins, ranging from 2 to 10 cm of diameter. On the other hand, MiNENs that include an acinar part as the non-endocrine component are more often nodular large neoplasms (4–8 cm in diameter), with more defined margins and the frequent presence of necrotic foci.[9] MiNEN can arise in all pancreatic districts and do not demonstrate any preference for a specific location.

MICROSCOPIC FEATURES

A classic example of MiNEN composed of NEC and ductal adenocarcinoma is represented in **Fig. 1**, whereas a classic example of MiNEN composed of NEC and acinar cell carcinoma is represented in **Fig. 2**.

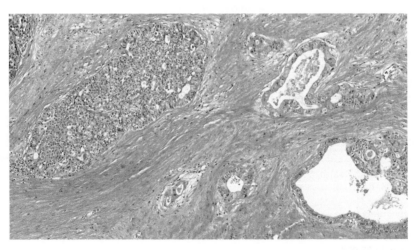

Fig. 1. Pancreatic MiNEN composed of neuroendocrine carcinoma (on the left) and ductal adenocarcinoma (on the right) (Hematoxylin-eosin, original magnification: 20x).

Fig. 2. Pancreatic MiNEN composed of neuroendocrine carcinoma (upper portion) and acinar cell carcinoma (lower portion). (Hematoxylin-eosin, original magnification: 10x).

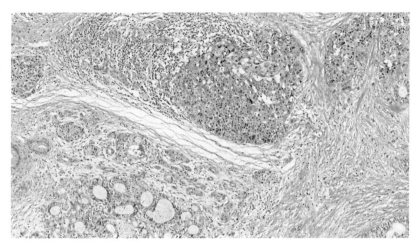

The diagnosis of MiNEN requires an in-depth comprehension of the morphologic aspects that characterize these mixed neoplasms and should respect some strict criteria (**Box 1**). All neoplasms classified as MiNEN are composed of at least two different components: non-endocrine (ductal adenocarcinoma and/or acinar cell carcinoma) and endocrine component (NEC or NET), both representing at least 30% of the tumor mass. The different components must be morphologically recognizable, and immunohistochemistry (IHC) is used for further confirmation of the morphologic diagnosis, but cannot be used alone. Indeed, as also recommended by the 2019 WHO classification, if a type of differentiation can be identified only by IHC, this situation does not fall into MiNEN category, where each component must be clearly identified first by histology. Both components, endocrine and non-endocrine, should be separately graded.[9]

The correct diagnosis along with a clear identification of each components and tumor grading is of importance also for guiding tumor staging and therapeutic approaches. MiNENs represent a heterogeneous group of neoplasms and their biological behavior depends indeed on the specific nature of their components. The neuroendocrine part is more often represented by poorly differentiated NEC, which can be composed of small or large cells. Small cell NECs are characterized by sheets of roundish, small cells with scant cytoplasm, and granular chromatin, with the presence of nuclear molding. On the other hand, large cell NECs, the most common subtype, are composed of large and round to polygonal cells with coarse chromatin and prominent nuclei. NECs are highly malignant neoplasms and show very often microscopic features representative of an aggressive biological behavior, such as vascular invasion (**Fig. 3**), necrosis, and perineural invasion. Of

---

Box 1
Diagnostic criteria for the diagnosis of pancreatic mixed neuroendocrine-non-neuroendocrine neoplasms and essential information to be reported into the final pathology report

Identifying the two separate components of the neoplasm.

- Endocrine component (NEC or NET)

- Malignant non-endocrine component (ductal adenocarcinoma or acinar cell carcinoma)

Each component must represent at least 30% of the tumor mass; in the pathology report, such percentages should be indicated

Both components should be morphologically recognizable

At least one of these classical IHC markers is mandatory to demonstrate with IHC the endocrine differentiation of the neuroendocrine component

- Synaptophysin

- Chromogranin A

Abbreviations: IHC, immunohistochemistry; NEC, neuroendocrine carcinoma; NET, neuroendocrine tumor.

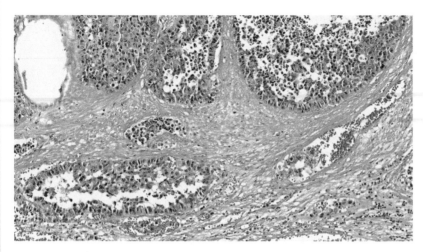

Fig. 3. Vascular invasion of the neuroendocrine component (neuroendocrine carcinoma) of a pancreatic MiNEN (Hematoxylin-eosin, original magnification: 20x). This is a common feature in this type of neoplasms, highlighting their highly malignant potential.

note, the neuroendocrine component can be represented also by pancreatic NET, which usually is nonfunctional NET.

Because of the limited data available in the literature on MiNEN cytology, there are still no established criteria for the diagnosis of MiNEN on cytologic smears. However, there are some published clinical cases with cytologic diagnosis of MiNEN.[10,11] In all such cytologic reports, fine-needle aspiration smears are described as hypercellular specimens, with cells single distributed or grouped in poorly cohesive clusters, with prominent nuclei with salt and pepper chromatin, positive for cytokeratin (CK) AE1/AE3, chromogranin A, and synaptophysin stains at the immunocytochemical level.[10,11] However, it has to be noted that, as indicated for histology, MiNENs represent a heterogeneous tumor entity, thus no definitive criteria independent from neoplastic components can exist. However, cytologic analysis can be considered as a potentially important tool to be considered into the multidisciplinary diagnostic process. The most important role of cytology in the case of MiNEN is to indicate the potential presence of a mixed neoplasm, as the definitive diagnosis can be reached only by histology, with a clear documentation of the presence of at least two tumor components, along with their quantification.

Although well-established histologic evidences and knowledge, the pathogenesis of MiNEN is still not well understood. The biphasic morphology of this tumor group could be explained with two main theories. According to some investigators, MiNENs are the result of the proliferation of two separate clones (collision tumors), and this may be true above all in the case of well differentiated NET as the neuroendocrine component; according to others, they arise from clonal evolution of either neuroendocrine line or from adenocarcinoma, and this is a widely accepted hypothesis above all in the case of NEC as the neuroendocrine component. Along this line, some molecular investigations provided robust indications that MiNEN (with NEC) can arise from a common precursor stem cell.[9,12]

DIFFERENTIAL DIAGNOSIS

The most important differential diagnosis and its most helpful tool along this line have been summarized in **Table 2**.

The main differential diagnoses of MiNEN regard their defining criteria and composition: indeed, in the case of a mixed neoplasm, the first aspect to be clarified is to obtain a reliable estimation of each single component. Indeed, if a component is less than 30% of the entire tumor mass, the neoplasm does not satisfy the diagnostic criteria of MiNEN and should be classified within the category of the largest tumor part, indicating that it has "aspects" or "features" of differentiation of the other component. For example, a pancreatic NEC with a 10% of acinar cell carcinoma should be classified as an NEC with acinar aspects.

Furthermore, the only IHC is not sufficient to support a diagnosis of MiNEN: for example, an acinar cell carcinoma with only immunohistochemical aspects of neuroendocrine differentiation, without any distinct morphologic patterns supporting the presence of this component, does not satisfy the criteria for MiNEN diagnosis and should be classified in the category of acinar cell carcinoma.

MiNENs that include a component of ductal adenocarcinoma should be distinguished from NET or NEC with entrapped normal ductules or

Table 2
Differential diagnosis

MiNEN VS.	Most Important Criteria for the Differential Diagnosis
Mixed neoplasm but not-MiNEN	The second component is <30% of the entire tumor mass. In this case, the neoplasm should be diagnosed in the category of the most represented tumor, adding "with aspects of [...]" for indicating the presence of another tumor component.
Not-real MiNEN, (1): IHC	If there is only IHC evidence of a second tumor differentiation, without a distinguished histologic criterion, this tumor cannot be classified as MiNEN.
Not-real MiNEN, (2): normal tissue	A ductal adenocarcinoma with entrapped normal islet or the NET/NEC with entrapped normal ductules/acinar parenchyma must be distinguished from MiNEN, first of all based the pure morphology.
Not-real MiNEN, (3): amphicrine neoplasms	Amphicrine neoplasms are not real MiNEN: they are composed of cells demonstrating at the same time both neuroendocrine and exocrine differentiation.
Not-real MiNEN, (4): MANET	The so-called MANET is mixed neoplasm composed of adenomatous non-endocrine and neuroendocrine components. The presence of an adenomatous component does not show any clinical implication, and thus the neuroendocrine component is the only clinically relevant.
Pancreatoblastoma	Pancreatoblastoma may resemble mixed neoplasms due to the presence of squamoid corpuscles. The most important point for the differential diagnosis with MiNEN is that they do not show neuroendocrine differentiation.

Abbreviations: MiNEN, Mixed neuroendocrine-non-neuroendocrine neoplasm; IHC, immunohistochemistry; NET, neuroendocrine tumor; NEC, neuroendocrine carcinoma.

acinar parenchyma or vice versa, from ductal adenocarcinoma with entrapped normal islets.

Another tumor entity, which could represent another differential diagnosis with MINEN, is represented by pancreatoblastoma, a neoplasm with acinar differentiation that includes squamous bodies, a microscopic feature that can be misinterpreted as mixed neoplasm. The most important criterion to differentiate MiNEN from pancreatoblastoma lies in the fact that the latter does not present a neuroendocrine differentiation; along the line of differential diagnosis, the presence of squamoid corpuscles in pancreatoblastoma represents another significant aspect.[13,14]

The last entities to complete the framework of MiNEN differential diagnosis are represented by amphicrine neoplasms, which are composed of cells simultaneously demonstrating both neuroendocrine and exocrine differentiation,[15–17] and by the so-called mixed adeno-neuroendocrine tumors (MANETs), which represent mixed neoplasms, composed of a neuroendocrine part mixed with an adenomatous non-endocrine component.[18–20] The correct identification of MANET lies in the fact that the presence of an adenomatous part does not impact the prognosis, which is influenced only by the neuroendocrine component.[18]

DIAGNOSIS

As already specified in different sections, the diagnosis of MiNEN requires the presence of at least two distinct entities, one neuroendocrine (NEC or, more rarely NET) and one ductal and/or acinar; such component must represent at least 30% of the entire tumor mass.

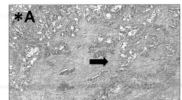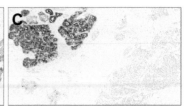

Fig. 4. Pancreatic MiNEN composed of neuroendocrine carcinoma (left part, indicated by a *black arrow*) and acinar cell carcinoma (on the left, *asterisk*). (*A*) Hematoxylin-eosin; (*B*) Synaptophysin; (*C*) Bcl-10; original magnification: 4x.

Of note, to be diagnosed as MiNEN both components of the neoplasia must be morphologically recognizable on hematoxylin-eosin slides, and the neuroendocrine component must stain positively the classical neuroendocrine markers synaptophysin and/or chromogranin A. Remaining on the immunohistochemical level, the non-endocrine component will be positive for the wide spectrum cytokeratin (CK8/18), carcinoembryonic antigen (CEA), and mucin 1 (MUC1) in the case of ductal differentiation, or Bcl-10 and trypsin in the case of acinar differentiation. A classical case of pancreatic MiNEN, along with IHC for synaptophysin and Bcl-10, is represented in **Fig. 4**.

Another essential IHC marker that should be always investigated for finalizing the diagnosis of MiNEN is the proliferative index Ki67. As also indicated in the last WHO classification, both MiNEN components should be graded separately. Along this line, Ki67 staining is a mandatory step for grading the neuroendocrine component. The proliferation grade in the NET component (Grades 1–3) is based on Ki67 nuclear staining and/or the number of mitotic figures counted on 2 mm² field (G1 <2 mitosis/2 mm² and Ki67 < 3%; G2: 2–20 mitosis/2 mm² and Ki67 3%–20%; G3: >20 mitosis/2 mm² and Ki67 > 20%). NECs have always a Ki67 index greater than 20% and are considered by definition as G3/high grade tumors (9). Interestingly, Milione and colleagues[12] demonstrated that Ki67 expression in the neuroendocrine component is the most reliable prognostic parameter, further corroborating the importance of its determination during routine diagnostic activity.

To further point out another important point regarding MiNEN diagnosis and IHC, it is of importance to note that relying only on IHC for MiNEN diagnosis is totally misleading. Some MiNEN indeed, and above all those with an acinar part as the non-endocrine component frequently express overlapping IHC features with NET/NEC. This could lead to misdiagnosis and not proper therapeutic approaches.

MOLECULAR PATHOLOGY FEATURES

The molecular features of MiNEN recapitulate the genetic profiles of tumor components. Indeed, in the case of ductal adenocarcinoma, the neoplasm will harbor the classic molecular alterations of this tumor type, including *KRAS*, *TP53*, and *SMAD4* mutations. At the same time, the presence of an acinar component will be highlighted by the presence of adenomatous polyposis coli (APC)/beta-catenin pathway alterations and *BRAF* fusions.[1,9] Regarding the neuroendocrine counterpart, since most of the cases display the NEC nature, the most common alterations in this setting regard those affecting *TP53* and *RB1*.[1,9] Current evidences on MiNEN biology, even if not pancreatic, support the monoclonal origin at least for MiNEN with NEC representing the neuroendocrine component.[1,9]

PROGNOSIS

During the years, the concept of pancreatic mixed tumors has evolved. Following the indications of the last WHO classification, only biphasic tumors composed of at least two morphologically recognizable neuroendocrine (constant) and non-endocrine (ductal and/or acinar) components satisfy this classification. The specific morphologic and immunohistochemical characteristics of MiNEN require particular attention from the oncologists to identify the most appropriate therapeutic regimen, which must take into account the tumor composition.

Of note, both MiNEN components of the tumor may display a combined but also an independent biological progression, and the metastatic disease can reflect only one of the two components. This vision indicates that the biological behavior of MiNEN does not represent the "mean value" between the two components, but the sum.[17,20,21] In this scenario, predicting the prognosis of MiNEN is very challenging. The most poorly differentiated/most aggressive component is more likely to

Box 2
Pitfalls box. Diagnostic pitfalls box

Entity Definition	Mixed Neoplasms That Do Not Satisfy the Diagnostic Criteria Are Not Classifiable as MiNEN
Normal tissue	Normal tissue (islets in PDAC or ducts/ductules/acinar parenchyma in NET/NEC) must be recognized by histology.
Neoadjuvant setting	MiNEN after chemotherapy must be assessed only in very selected cases, acknowledging that tissue modification after CT are still largely unknown.

Abbreviations: CT, chemotherapy; MiNEN, mixed neuroendocrine-non-neuroendocrine neoplasm; NEC, neuroendocrine carcinoma; NET, neuroendocrine tumor; PDAC, pancreatic ductal adenocarcinoma.

determine the general clinical course. Along this line, patients with ductal non-endocrine component have relatively poor prognosis, similar to those affected by pure conventional adenocarcinoma.[9] Similarly, patients with an acinar component may demonstrate the same prognosis as patients with pure acinar carcinomas, with 5-year survival rate ranging from 30% to 50%.[1,9] In these cases, however, the presence of an associated NEC is more likely to drive the prognosis toward a more malignant behavior. In cases where a NET represents the neuroendocrine component, the prognosis is determined by the non-endocrine component. All these observations further highlight the pivotal role of pathologists for a correct diagnosis of MiNEN.

be histologically recognizable. The neuroendocrine part is always present. The diagnosis of MiNEN is based on morphology, but a specific IHC is required for confirming the nature of the neoplasm. The constant neuroendocrine component, which is more often represented by NEC, is positive for synaptophysin and/or chromogranin A, the eventual ductal component is positive for cytokeratin 7, 8/18, and MUC1, and the eventual acinar component is positive for Bcl-10 and trypsin.[1,9] The main molecular alterations reflect those of each part. Also, the prognosis of MiNEN is very heterogeneous and depends on the different tumor components; of note, the more aggressive tumor part drives the clinical course.

SUMMARY

Pancreatic MiNENs are rare neoplasms, composed of at least two components that must

CLINICS CARE POINTS/DIAGNOSTIC PITFALLS

The most important diagnostic pitfalls are summarized in *Pitfalls box* (**Box 2**).

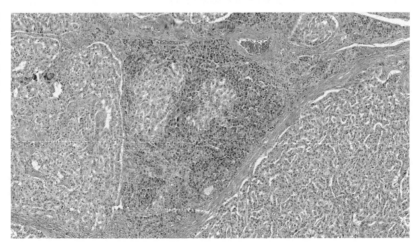

Fig. 5. Entrapped acini in a pancreatic neuroendocrine tumor (hematoxylin-eosin, original magnification: 20x). This feature represents a potential diagnostic pitfall for MiNEN.

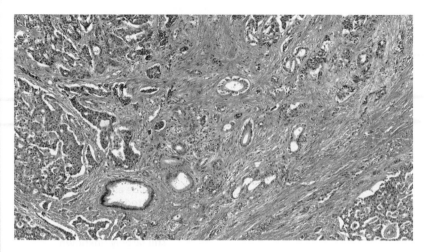

Fig. 6. Entrapped ductules in a pancreatic neuroendocrine tumor (hematoxylin-eosin, original magnification: 20x). This feature represents a potential diagnostic pitfall for MiNEN.

The first diagnostic pitfall regards biphasic tumors that do not satisfy the requirement for MiNEN diagnosis, as also specified in the section on differential diagnosis. Along this line, the most important points are (i) reaching the threshold of at least 30% of the tumor mass and (ii) the possibility of a morphologic distinction of each component, because IHC alone is not an accepted criterion for MiNEN diagnosis.

Other possible pitfalls regard the histologic recognition of normal tissue entrapped within the tumor mass. Indeed, normal islets entrapped in a ductal adenocarcinoma or, conversely, normal acini (**Fig. 5**) or normal ducts/ductules (**Fig. 6**) entrapped in a neuroendocrine neoplasm may mimic a mixed tumor. In such cases, the distinction should be based on histologic criteria, although IHC in this situation does not represent a helpful tool.

The last important diagnostic pitfall regards the diagnosis of MiNEN after chemotherapy. Indeed, it is still largely unknown what is the exact role of chemotherapy in influencing tumor morphology. Along this line, various investigators published data on the increased number of neuroendocrine cells in the neo-adjuvant setting; one hypothesis for this phenomenon is that neuroendocrine cells are terminally differentiated, less-proliferating and thus less responsive to chemotherapy, as also observed in pancreas and other organs.[22–25] This indicates that the possibility of an MiNEN diagnosis in the neo-adjuvant setting should be considered in very selected cases.

DISCLOSURE

The authors have nothing to disclose.

REFERENCES

1. Lloyd RV, Osamura RY, Kloppel G, et al, editors. World Health Organization classification of tumors of endocrine organs. 4th Edition. Lyon: IARC Press; 2017.
2. Reid MD, Akkas G, Basturk O, et al. Mixed adenoneuroendocrine carcinoma of the pancreas. In: La Rosa S, Sessa F, editors. Pancreatic neuroendocrine neoplasms: practical approach to diagnosis classification, and therapy. New York: Springer; 2015. p. 155–65.
3. Klimstra DS, Rosai J, Heffess CS. Mixed acinar-endocrine carcinomas of the pancreas. Am J Surg Pathol 1994;18:765–78.
4. La Rosa S, Adsay V, Albarello L, et al. Clinicopathologic study of 62 acinar cell carcinomas of the pancreas: insights into the morphology and immunophenotype and search for prognostic markers. Am J Surg Pathol 2012;36:1782–95.
5. Lewin K. Carcinoid tumors and the mixed (composite) glandular-endocrine cell carcinomas. Am J Surg Pathol 1987;11(Suppl. 1):71–86.
6. Capella C, La Rosa S, Uccella S, et al. Mixed endocrine-exocrine tumors of the gastrointestinal tract. Semin Diagn Pathol 2000;17:91–103.
7. Solcia E, Kloppel G, Sobin LH, et al. Histological typing of endocrine tumours. Heidelberg: Springer-Verlag; 2000.
8. Bosman FT, Carneiro F, Hruban RH, et al, editors. World Health Organization classification of tumors of the digestive system. 4th edition. Lyon: IARC Press; 2010.
9. World Health Organization Classification of Tumors Editorial Board. In: World Health Organization classification of tumors. Digestive system tumors. 5th edition. Lyon: IARC Press; 2019.
10. Strait AM, Sharma N, Tsapakos MJ, et al. Pancreatic mixed acinar-neuroendocrine carcinoma, a unique diagnostic challenge on FNA cytology: A small

series of two cases with literature review. Diagn Cytopathol 2018;46:971–6.

11. Lee L, Bajor-Dattilo EB, Das K. Metastatic mixed acinar-neuroendocrine carcinoma of the pancreas to the liver: a cytopathology case report with review of the literature. Diagn Cytopathol 2013;41:164–70.

12. Milione M, Maisonneuve P, Pellegrinelli A, et al. Ki67 proliferative index of the neuroendocrine component drives MANEC prognosis. Endocr Relat Cancer 2018;25:583–93.

13. Salman B, Brat G, Yoon YS, et al. The diagnosis and surgical treatment of pancreatoblastoma in adults: a case series and review of the literature. J Gastrointest Surg 2013;17:2153–61.

14. Luchini C, Pelosi G, Scarpa A, et al. Neuroendocrine neoplasms of the biliary tree, liver and pancreas: a pathological approach. Pathologica 2021;113:28–38.

15. Akki AS, Liu X, Clapp WL, et al. Mixed acinar-neuroendocrine carcinoma with amphicrine features of the pancreas: Two rare cases with diffuse co-expression of acinar and neuroendocrine markers. Pathol Int 2021;71(7):485–7. Epub ahead of print.

16. Ratzenhofer M, Aubock L. The amphicrine (endo-exocrine) cells in the human gut, with a short reference to amphicrine neoplasias. Acta Morphol Acad Sci Hung 1980;28:37–58.

17. Uccella S, La Rosa S. Looking into digestive mixed neuroendocrine - nonneuroendocrine neoplasms: subtypes, prognosis, and predictive factors. Histopathology 2020;77:700–17.

18. La Rosa S, Uccella S, Molinari F, et al. Mixed adenoma well-differentiated neuroendocrine tumor (MANET) of the digestive system: an indolent subtype of mixed neuroendocrine-nonneuroendocrine neoplasm (MiNEN). Am J Surg Pathol 2018;42: 1503–12.

19. Huang D, Ren F, Ni S, et al. Amphicrine carcinoma of the stomach and intestine: a clinicopathologic and pan-cancer transcriptome analysis of a distinct entity. Cancer Cell Int 2019;19:310.

20. de Mestier L, Cros J, Neuzillet C, et al. Digestive system mixed neuroendocrine-non-neuroendocrine neoplasms. Neuroendocrinology 2017;105:412–25.

21. Frizziero M, Chakrabarty B, Nagy B, et al. Mixed neuroendocrine non-neuroendocrine neoplasms: a systematic review of a controversial and underestimated diagnosis. J Clin Med 2020;9:273.

22. Shia J, Tickoo SK, Guillem JG, et al. Increased endocrine cells in treated rectal adenocarcinomas: a possible reflection of endocrine differentiation in tumor cells induced by chemotherapy and radiotherapy. Am J Surg Pathol 2002;26:863–72.

23. Oneda E, Liserre B, Bianchi D, et al. Diagnosis of mixed adenoneuroendocrine carcinoma (MANEC) after neoadjuvant chemotherapy for pancreatic and gastric adenocarcinoma: two case reports and a review of the literature. Case Rep Oncol 2019;12: 434–42.

24. Spiotto MT, Chung TD. STAT3 mediates IL-6-induced neuroendocrine differentiation in prostate cancer cells. Prostate 2000;42:186–95.

25. Terry S, Beltran H. The many faces of neuroendocrine differentiation in prostate cancer progression. Front Oncol 2014;4:60.

The Clinical and Pathologic Features of Intracholecystic Papillary-Tubular Neoplasms of the Gallbladder

Heba Abdelal, MD[a], Deyali Chatterjee, MD[b],*

KEYWORDS

- Intracholecystic papillary-tubular neoplasm • Intracholecystic papillary neoplasm • Gallbladder
- ICPN

Key points

- ICPN is a demarcated mucosal-based exophytic neoplastic lesion involving the gallbladder.
- ICPN may be associated with invasive carcinoma.
- The prognosis of ICPN-associated invasive carcinoma is much better than conventional gallbladder carcinoma.
- ICPN also shows association with background flat dysplasia in the gallbladder and a field effect in the biliary tree, rendering the patient susceptible to subsequent development of biliary tract cancer arising at another site.
- Other polypoid lesions (benign or nonneoplastic) need to be distinguished from ICPN, as the malignant potentials of these entities are vastly different.
- The pathology of ICPN may be challenging because it involves a variety of epithelial subtypes, architectural patterns, and histologic variations in the invasive carcinoma component.

Abbreviations

ICPN	Intracholecystic papillary-tubular neoplasm

ABSTRACT

Intracholecystic papillary-tubular neoplasm denotes a discrete mucosal-based neoplastic proliferation into the gallbladder lumen. It is diagnosed incidentally during cholecystectomy or radiologically during a workup for abdominal pain. The majority of polypoid lesions in the gallbladder are non-neoplastic; therefore, pathologic examination is the gold standard to establish this diagnosis. Intracholecystic papillary-tubular neoplasm is considered as premalignant, although associated invasive carcinomas may be present in the specimen. Invasive carcinoma arising from intracholecystic papillary-tubular neoplasm have a better prognosis than de novo gallbladder carcinomas. The pathology of intracholecystic papillary-tubular neoplasm, including the challenges involved in the diagnosis of this entity, is discussed.

[a] Department of Pathology, Yale School of Medicine, 310 Cedar Street, New Haven, CT, USA; [b] Department of Pathology, The University of Texas MD Anderson Cancer Center, 1515 Holcombe Boulevard, Houston, TX 77030, USA
* Corresponding author.
E-mail address: Dchatterjee@mdanderson.org

Surgical Pathology 15 (2022) 565–577
https://doi.org/10.1016/j.path.2022.05.011
1875-9181/22/© 2022 Elsevier Inc. All rights reserved.

OVERVIEW

According to the current World Health Organization (WHO) classification, benign or premalignant epithelial tumors of the gallbladder forming a grossly visible, mucosal-based lesion that projects into the lumen without histologic evidence of invasion, are interchangeably referred to as intracholecystic papillary-tubular neoplasm or intracholecystic papillary neoplasm, both abbreviated as ICPN. When invasive carcinoma is associated with such a lesion, it is classified as ICPN with associated invasive carcinoma.

A size criteria of 1 cm was originally suggested arbitrarily by authors who coined the term ICPN.[1] This nomenclature was based on the size criteria used for pancreatic intraductal papillary mucinous neoplasms (IPMN) to include this entity in the same spectrum, and also based on the general observation that usually larger lesions were associated with invasive carcinoma. The current fifth edition of the WHO Digestive System Tumors has not included a size criteria for this group of neoplasms.[2]

DEMOGRAPHIC FEATURES

The reported incidence among cholecystectomy cases varies in different studies, lower in Eastern literature than from the West (0.4%–4.0%).[1,3] These studies have also reported variation in the incidence of gallbladder cancer arising in association with ICPN. Approximately 20% have been reported to be associated with gallstones[1]/chronic cholecystitis. ICPN is more common in females.[3] They are almost exclusively reported in adults (age range, 20–94 years; mean, 61 years).[1]

SYMPTOMATOLOGY AND PREOPERATIVE EVALUATION

Patients are symptomatic in only 50% of the cases, and present with right upper quadrant pain.[1] The remaining cases are asymptomatic. A subset of the latter undergo cholecystectomy for incidental detection of a polypoid lesion in the gallbladder on imaging. Currently, cholecystectomy is generally not advocated for polypoid lesions less than 1 cm in the absence of symptoms, although this is also considered to be an insensitive parameter and radiologic distinction between neoplastic and non-neoplastic nature of the polyps are being investigated as alternative to providing a surgical management decision.[4,5]

GROSS FEATURES

ICPN presents with an exophytic intraluminal growth (Fig. 1), with a lobulated or granular or filiform surface, and may be friable. Some are pedunculated and others have a broad base (sessile). Approximately one-third of cases are reported to be multifocal. Tumors may arise anywhere in the gallbladder, including the neck, but have been reported more commonly in the fundus and body.[3]

TUMOR SIZE

The average tumor size in the study that including a size criteria of 1.0 cm was reported as 2.2 cm (median).[1]

MICROSCOPIC FEATURES

ARCHITECTURE

Dense epithelial proliferation arranged in a papillary (Fig. 2A, B), tubular (Fig. 3A, B), or tubulopapillary (Fig. 4A, B) configuration, often appearing back to back with scant intervening stroma. These neoplasms grow exophytically into the lumen of the gallbladder, but may extend into the Rokitansky–Aschoff sinuses, and this needs to be distinguished from invasive adenocarcinoma. Rarely, they may arise only within Rokitansky–Aschoff sinuses without surface epithelial

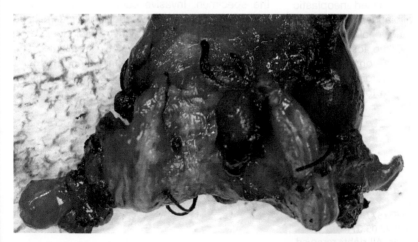

Fig. 1. Gross appearance of ICPN: sharply demarcated exophytic intraluminal growth. (gross image)

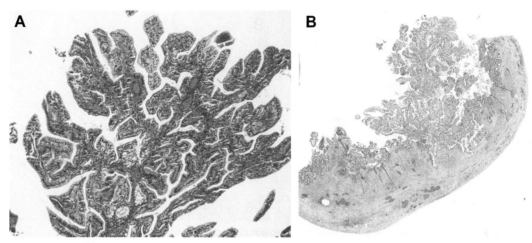

Fig. 2. (*A, B*) Papillary architecture of ICPN, 2 separate cases. (hematoxylin-eosin stain)

involvement.[6] There is also a rare possibility that the polypoid lesion may be located closer to the neck of the gallbladder and extend into the bile duct with the base still confined to gallbladder.[7]

EPITHELIAL SUBTYPES

ICPNs are often composed of a heterogeneous mixture of different epithelial subtypes. The epithelial cell types that are commonly identified in this lesion include biliary (Fig. 5A, B), gastric foveolar (Fig. 6A–C), gastric pyloric (Fig. 7A–D), intestinal (Fig. 8A, B), or other special types, such as oncocytic (Fig. 9) and clear cell (Fig. 10). The descriptives associated with these different epithelial subtypes are enumerated in Table 1. Often, there is a mixture of epithelial subtypes in the same neoplasm, although association with high-grade dysplasia and invasive carcinoma vary, depending on the epithelial subtype.[8]

The gastric pyloric subtype is recognized as a distinct subtype by the WHO and labeled as pyloric gland adenoma. This designation is supported by the features of being composed of a single epithelial type (as compared with other ICPNs, which usually show a mixed epithelial phenotype), usually tubular rather than papillary, smaller in size than other variants, and least likely to be associated with background flat dysplasia or with malignant transformation. However, malignant potential is not absent in these neoplasms, and high-grade dysplasia can also be observed. A separate nomenclature for these lesions (pyloric gland adenoma) is not justified.[9,10]

DYSPLASIA

The epithelium may seem bland and metaplastic type, but may also show low- and high-grade dysplasia based on cytoarchitectural features. By

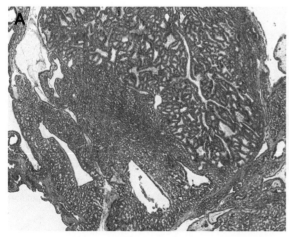

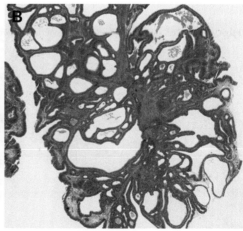

Fig. 3. (*A, B*) Tubular architecture of ICPN, 2 separate cases. (hematoxylin-eosin stain)

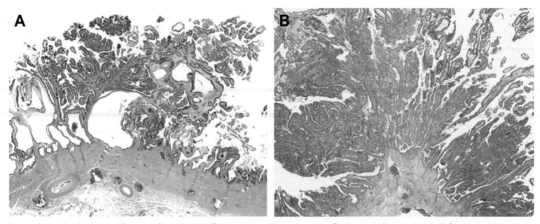

Fig. 4. (A, B) Tubulopapillary architecture of ICPN, 2 separate cases. (hematoxylin-eosin stain)

definition, all epithelial changes not cytologically high-grade dysplasia are considered as low-grade dysplasia. The distinction of cytologic low- and high-grade dysplasia is highlighted in **Table 2**. Invasive carcinoma correlates with the presence and extent of high-grade dysplasia in ICPN.[11]

BACKGROUND MUCOSA

Approximately one-half of the cases have been reported to be associated with background flat dysplasia (**Fig. 11**).

INTRACHOLECYSTIC PAPILLARY-TUBULAR NEOPLASM WITH ASSOCIATED INVASIVE CARCINOMA

This group of invasive carcinomas are reported to comprise approximately 6% of all gallbladder carcinomas in 1 report (**Fig. 12**A–C).[1] The majority of these carcinomas are adenocarcinoma (cholangiocarcinoma), but other rare tumor types such as adenosquamous and squamous cell carcinoma, neuroendocrine carcinoma, mixed neuroendocrine–non-neuroendocrine neoplasm, medullary, signet ring, and sarcomatoid carcinoma may be seen.[12–14] There is no demographic difference between ICPN cases with or without invasion, but invasive carcinoma is more commonly seen in larger ICPN, with papillary architecture rather than tubular, and most frequently associated with the biliary epithelial subtype, as well as correlates with the extent of high-grade dysplasia, reinforcing the adenoma–carcinoma sequence that is a feature throughout the gastrointestinal and pancreatobiliary tract. Invasive carcinoma is identified by the haphazard arrangement of neoplastic glands within the wall of the gallbladder near the base of the ICPN, usually associated with a desmoplastic stromal response. When areas of poorer differentiation in an adenocarcinoma, such as single infiltrative neoplastic cells or abortive glands are identified, the diagnosis of an associated invasive component is easy, but in the context of a well-differentiated adenocarcinoma, careful

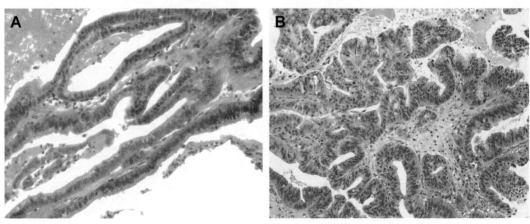

Fig. 5. Biliary epithelial subtype in ICPN. (A) Low-grade dysplasia. (B) High-grade dysplasia. (hematoxylin-eosin stain).

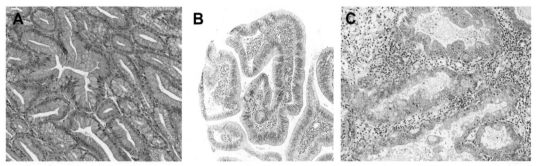

Fig. 6. Gastric foveolar epithelial subtype in ICPN. (*A*) Bland epithelium, by definition, low-grade dysplasia. (*B*) Cytologic low-grade dysplasia. (*C*) High-grade dysplasia. (hematoxylin-eosin stain).

distinction from extension into Rokitansky–Aschoff sinuses need to be made.

MOLECULAR FEATURES

Not much is known about the molecular pathway of ICPNs. Recently, analysis from the Cancer Genome Atlas database showed 6 genes (FGA, CFH, ENPP1, CFHR3, ITIH4, and NAT2) to be highly expressed in gallbladder cancer and significantly correlated with worse prognosis.[15] How carcinoma associated with ICPN compares to de novo gallbladder cancer is currently not known. KRAS and TP53 mutations, which are common in intraductal papillary-tubular neoplasm of the bile duct and IPMN, has rarely been reported in ICPN. However, p53 alterations have been reported in tumors with a neuroendocrine carcinoma as the invasive component.[16,17]

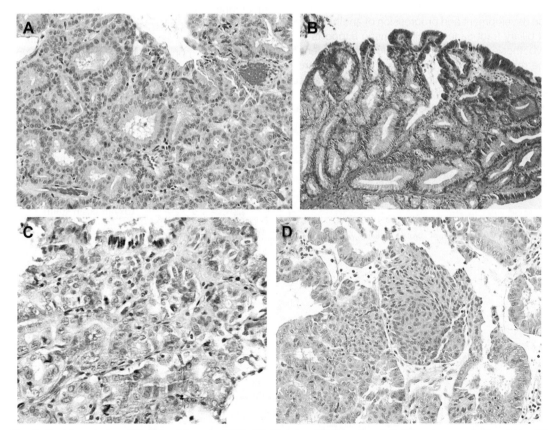

Fig. 7. Gastric pyloric epithelial subtype in ICPN. (*A*) Bland epithelium, by definition, low-grade dysplasia. (*B*) Cytologic low-grade dysplasia. (*C*) High-grade dysplasia. (*D*) With squamoid morule. (hematoxylin-eosin stain).

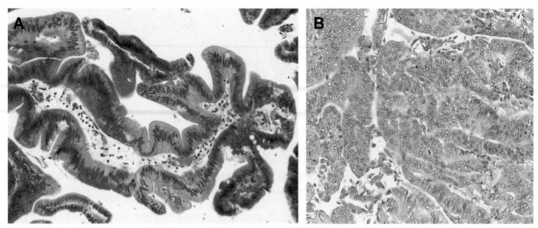

Fig. 8. Intestinal epithelial subtype in ICPN. (A) Low-grade dysplasia. (B) High-grade dysplasia. (hematoxylin-eosin stain).

PROGNOSIS

A stage-matched comparison of carcinoma arising in ICPN and those without showed a significant survival advantage in the former group.[1] Therefore, recognition of carcinoma arising in ICPN in the pathology report is of clinical importance. Survival of noninvasive ICPN is not at 100% owing to the development and progression of another focus of biliary tract cancer. This scenario supports the hypothesis that this is due to field effect rendering the remainder of the biliary tract at risk of carcinoma. Therefore, clinical follow-up is warranted after resection of ICPN.

DIFFERENTIAL DIAGNOSIS AND DIAGNOSTIC CHALLENGES

ICPN needs to be distinguished from benign polypoid lesions, such as cholesterol polyps, inflammatory polyps, adenomyomas, and polypoid metaplasia and hyperplasia (Fig. 13) in the setting of chronic cholecystitis.[18,19] The latter category has no malignant potential, in contrast with ICPNs. Although a true estimate of the proportion of neoplastic to non-neoplastic gallbladder polyps is lacking, a recent study has shown approximately half of gallbladder polyps to be neoplastic, and, compared with non-neoplastic polyps, these

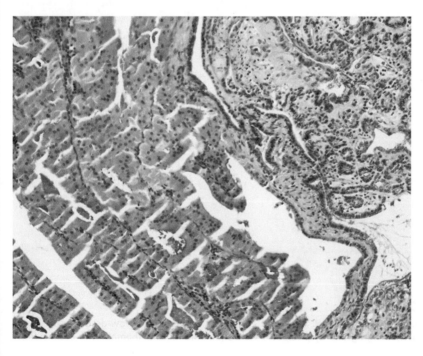

Fig. 9. Oncocytic epithelial subtype in ICPN (left side of the image, admixed with biliary type epithelium on the right side of the image). [hematoxylin-eosin stain]

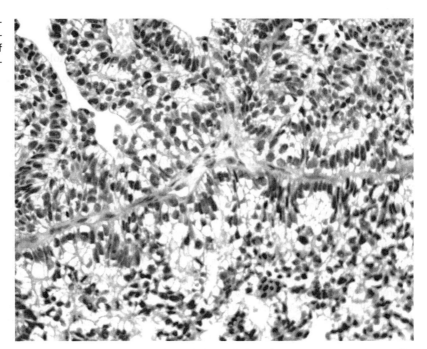

Fig. 10. Clear cell epithelial subtype in ICPN (regarded as a variant of biliary subtype). [hematoxylin-eosin stain]

were larger, more often single than multiple, more sessile than pedunculated, and had a greater association with gallstones.[5] Apart from cytoarchitectural features, non-neoplastic polypoid lesions may not be as sharply circumscribed from the background mucosa, as is usually seen in ICPN.

ICPN needs to be distinguished from biliary intraepithelial neoplasia, which is characterized by a flat or micropapillary appearance of dysplasia only recognized microscopically (vs ICPN, which has a grossly identifiable component). Although a size cutoff is not currently supported by the WHO, a microscopic focus of papillary architecture that does not have a macroscopic correlate should be placed into the biliary intraepithelial neoplasia category rather than ICPN (similar to the criteria used for pancreatic intraepithelial neoplasia vs IPMN in the pancreas). However, occasionally, there may be a morphologic continuum that may be observed between ICPN and background biliary intraepithelial neoplasia,[20] as illustrated in **Fig. 11**.

Distinction of ICPN extending into the Rokitansky–Aschoff sinuses from invasive carcinoma is of paramount importance. In the former context, it still qualifies as an in situ neoplasm. The Rokitansky–Aschoff sinuses are usually

Table 1
The descriptives associated with these different epithelial subtypes

Epithelial Type	Cytologic Description	Immunohistochemical Features
Intestinal	Pseudostratified columnar cells with elongated nuclei and basophilic cytoplasm, resembling colonic adenoma	MUC2, CDX2
Gastric foveolar	Tall columnar cells with abundant apical pale mucin, resembling gastric foveolar cells	MUC5AC
Gastric pyloric	Foamy mucinous cytoplasm in cuboidal to short columnar cells, resembling gastric pyloric glands; squamoid morules may be present	MUC6
Biliary	Nondescript cuboidal cells often with eosinophilic cytoplasm, resembling epithelium of the pancreatobiliary tract	MUC1
Other cell types	Clear cell features, intestinal-type columnar cells but with eosinophilic cytoplasm, oncocytic	

Table 2
The distinction of cytologic low- and high-grade dysplasia

Type of Dysplasia	Architecture	Cytology
Low grade	Simple papillary, tubular, tubulopapillary architecture	No or minimal atypia, to pseudostratification, but without loss of polarity (intestinal subtype)
High grade	Mostly tubulopapillary or papillary, with marked architectural complexity with disorganization, and gland-in-gland appearance	Nuclear stratification, loss of polarity, mucin depletion, variation in nuclear size and chromatin pattern

surrounded by smooth muscle hyperplasia. Abrupt transition of neoplastic epithelium and pre-existing epithelium may be identified,[3] and is helpful in the distinction (**Fig. 14**). In cases of invasive carcinoma, there will be associated inflammatory and desmoplastic reaction, and, unless very well-differentiated adenocarcinoma, poorly formed or abortive glands or single cells may be identified, as illustrated in **Fig. 12C**.

Adenocarcinoma may show surface papillary components (**Fig. 15**) and this feature should not be misinterpreted as ICPN. In the former setting, a discrete intraluminal growth with a defined base and distinct from adjacent mucosa is usually not identified. Invasive adenocarcinoma may be present elsewhere from the location of ICPN (**Fig. 16**). This scenario is not clearly stated in the current literature and may cause a diagnostic dilemma. Based on the current definition of the entities, a diagnosis of conventional adenocarcinoma arising from background high-grade flat dysplasia in the gallbladder, along with a simultaneous noninvasive ICPN, is favored over labeling this as ICPN with associated invasive carcinoma.

When an ICPN is much smaller than the size of invasive adenocarcinoma (**Fig. 17**), it is not clear whether this represents an ICPN associated with invasive carcinoma or a conventional gallbladder adenocarcinoma with focal surface exophytic component. Reporting this entity descriptively in the section for comment or microscopic description may be helpful based on the current level of understanding.

SPECIAL PRECAUTIONS TO BE TAKEN DURING PATHOLOGIC EXAMINATION

A. Careful examination of the luminal contents of the gallbladder need to be done routinely, because some pendunculated ICPNs can become detached and float within the lumen.
B. A grossly identifiable mucosal based lesion regardless of size (ICPN) needs to be entirely submitted for histologic evaluation, unless

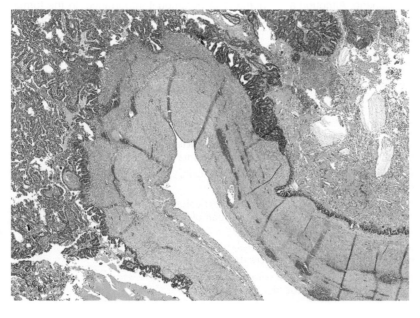

Fig. 11. Background flat dysplasia associated with IPMN. (hematoxylin-eosin stain)

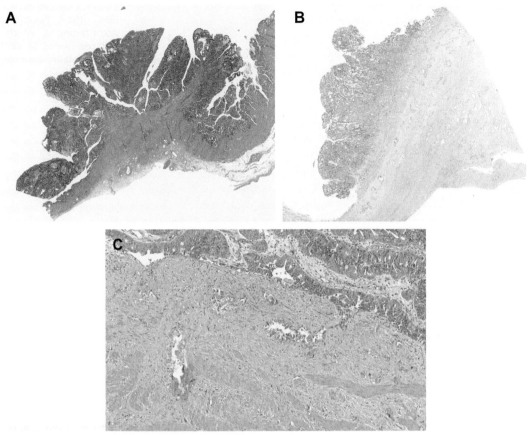

Fig. 12. ICPN with associated invasive carcinoma. (A) Focal invasion. (B) Extensive invasion. (C) Features of invasive adenocarcinoma, manifested by haphazard arrangement of glands in the underlying stroma, single cells or abortive glands, and stromal desmoplastic reaction. (hematoxylin-eosin stain).

Fig. 13. Polypoid hyperplasia in chronic cholecystitis, a non-neoplastic condition that can mimic ICPN. (hematoxylin-eosin stain)

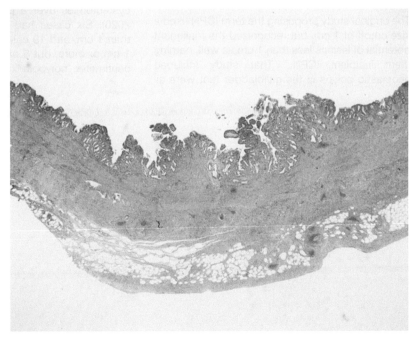

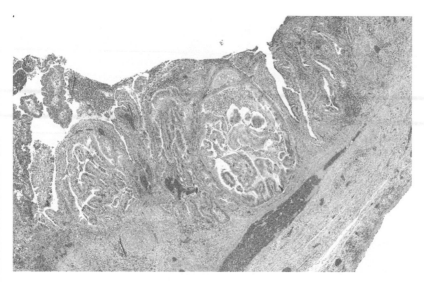

Fig. 14. Extension of ICPN into the Rokitansky–Aschoff sinuses, which is still considered as an in situ neoplasm. (hematoxylin-eosin stain)

there is a gross suggestion of invasive carcinoma within the specimen.

C. If there is no invasive carcinoma associated with an identified ICPN, but there is background flat high-grade dysplasia, the entire gallbladder needs to be submitted to rule out invasive carcinoma which may be located away from the ICPN.

FUTURE DIRECTIONS

ESTABLISHING THE SIZE CRITERIA OF INTRACHOLECYSTIC PAPILLARY-TUBULAR NEOPLASM

The original study proposing the term ICPN used a size cutoff of 1 cm, but recognized the malignant potential of lesions less than 1 cm as well, naming them incipient ICPN.[1] That study included neoplastic polyps in the gallbladder that were all greater than 1 cm, so there was no scope to study the true malignant potential of smaller lesions. Although it is recognized that the malignant potential increases with increase in size of ICPN, a recent study has shown that a size cutoff of 10 mm is not justified; several of the polyps less than 10 mm were neoplastic in nature, and 1 polypoid lesion less than 10 mm showed invasive malignancy.[21] Confirming this finding is our own study (Heba Abdelal, MD, Deyali Chatterjee, MD, 2020) performed at a large tertiary care institution supported by the institutional review board. Briefly, a total of 25 neoplastic polyps were identified, all in adults (15 females, 10 males; mean age, 62 years) from a search database of 8723 cholecystectomies over a period of 25 years (2008–2020). Six cases had neoplastic polyps greater than 1 cm, and 19 cases (76%) had a polyp size 1 cm or more, but 5 of them had additional subcentimeter polypoid neoplastic lesions. Eleven

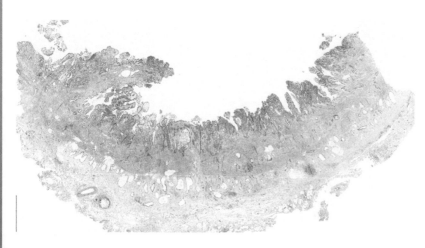

Fig. 15. Involvement of surface mucosa with some papillary configuration may be seen in conventional adenocarcinoma. (hematoxylin-eosin stain)

Fig. 16. Foci of invasive adenocarcinoma are present elsewhere in the gallbladder wall (marked on the slide imaged) associated with flat dysplasia, while simultaneously, there is an ICPN, which does not show invasive adenocarcinoma at the base of that lesion. (hematoxylin-eosin stain).

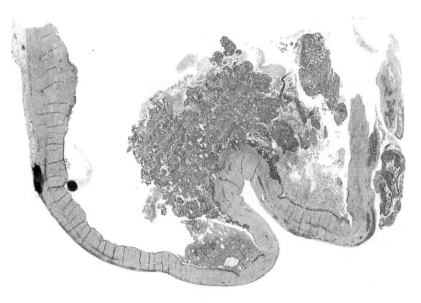

cases (44%) were symptomatic with right upper quadrant pain and imaging showed a gallbladder mass, whereas others were asymptomatic (8 cases were detected by radiology for other reasons and the rest were incidentally discovered at cholecystectomy). A clinicopathologic comparison of the groups are shown in **Table 3**. As expected, the incidence of high-grade dysplasia is apparently higher in neoplasms greater than 1 cm and associated invasive carcinoma were not seen in neoplasms less than 1 cm (only 6 cases were identified in this cohort, and the differences were not statistically significant using a χ^2 test and Fisher's exact test where applicable). There

were also no statistical differences between demographic features, multiplicity of lesions, clinical presentation, relevant disease associations such as cholelithiasis or primary sclerosing cholangitis, composition of epithelial cell types, or incidence of background flat dysplasia. Therefore, we support the hypothesis that subcentimeter polypoid lesions in gallbladder with papillary, tubular, or tubulopapillary growth, showing florid epithelial proliferation with scant stroma, are essentially neoplastic and in the same spectrum as ICPN. Morphologic recognition of this entity is needed and other benign or non-neoplastic mucosal polypoid lesions need to be excluded before

Fig. 17. The size of the gallbladder adenocarcinoma is much larger compared with the luminal exophytic component. (hematoxylin-eosin stain)

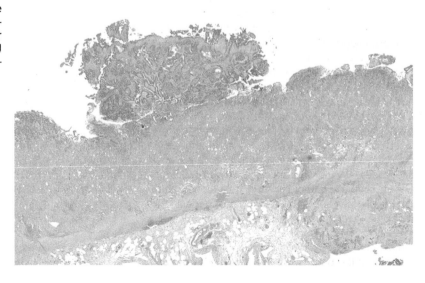

Table 3
A clinicopathologic comparison of the groups

Clinicopathologic Features	Polypoid Neoplasm <1 cm (n = 6)	Polypoid Neoplasm 1 cm or More (n = 19)
Average size, cm	0.4 (0.2–0.7)	2.3 (1–8.2)
Gender distribution	Female = 5, male = 1	Female = 10, male = 9
Age in years, mean (range)	59 (31–91)	63 (41–85)
Multiplicity of lesions	2 (33.3%)	6 (31.5%)
Clinical presentation (asymptomatic:symptomatic)	4:2	10:9
Multiplicity of epithelial components	2 (33.3%)	12 (63.1%)
Epithelial types (number of lesions involved)	Biliary (4) Gastric (3) Intestinal (1) Other: Clear cell change (1)	Biliary (17) Gastric (9) Intestinal (4) Other: Oncocytic (2)
Cytologic dysplasia	Cytologically bland (metaplastic type) – 3 (50%) Cytologic low-grade dysplasia – 1 (16.7%) High-grade dysplasia – 2 (33.3%)	Cytologically bland (metaplastic type) – 2 (10.5%) Cytologic low-grade dysplasia – 2 (10.5%) High-grade dysplasia –15 (78.9%)
Associated invasive carcinoma	0	7 (36.8%)
Background flat dysplasia	2 (33.3%) low grade	9 (56.3%) low grade: 6, high grade: 4
Association with cholelithiasis	3 (50%)	9 (47.3%)
Association with primary sclerosing cholangitis	1 (16.7%)	2 (10.5%)

labeling the lesion as ICPN, rather than using any size criteria.

UNIFICATION OF TERMINOLOGY

The term ICPN was introduced as a part of the same strategy to unify the concept of intramucosal neoplastic mass-forming neoplasms throughout the pancreatobiliary tract. However, there are subtle morphologic and molecular differences among these neoplasms, rendering a variety of terminology to specifically define these entities, ranging from IPMN, intraductal oncocytic papillary neoplasm and intraductal tubulopapillary neoplasm in the pancreas, to intraductal papillary–tubular neoplasm of bile ducts (subdivided into types 1 and 2[22]), intra-ampullary papillary–tubular neoplasm, and ICPN. These entities have several similarities and subtle differences in their pathologic manifestations. Not much is known about the spectrum of underlying molecular alterations, especially with any clinical relevance, and, as such, the varied terminologies remain confusing to most practicing pathologists and defeat the purpose of the recent changes in

nomenclature for the purpose of unification of these group of neoplasms.

DISCLOSURE

No commercial or financial conflicts of interest or any funding sources for all authors.

REFERENCES

1. Adsay V, Jang KT, Roa JC, et al. Intracholecystic papillary-tubular neoplasms (ICPN) of the gallbladder (neoplastic polyps, adenomas, and papillary neoplasms that are ≥1.0 cm): clinicopathologic and immunohistochemical analysis of 123 cases. Am J Surg Pathol 2012;36(9): 1279–301.

2. Basturk OAS, Esposito I. Intracholecystic papillary neoplasm. In: WHO Classification of Tumours Editorial Board, editor. Digestive System Tumours, vol. 1, 5th edition. Lyon (France): International Agency for Research on Cancer; 2019. p. 276–8.

3. Nakanuma Y, Nomura Y, Watanabe H, et al. Pathological characterization of intracholecystic papillary neoplasm: a recently proposed preinvasive neoplasm of gallbladder. Ann Diagn Pathol 2021;52:151723.

4. Yin SN, Shen GH, Liu L, et al. Triphasic dynamic enhanced computed tomography for differentiating cholesterol and adenomatous gallbladder polyps. Abdom Radiol (NY) 2021;46(10):4701–8.

5. Wennmacker SZ, van Dijk AH, Raessens JHJ, et al. Polyp size of 1 cm is insufficient to discriminate neoplastic and non-neoplastic gallbladder polyps. Surg Endosc 2019;33(5):1564–71.

6. Muranushi R, Saito H, Matsumoto A, et al. A case report of intracholecystic papillary neoplasm of the gallbladder resembling a submucosal tumor. Surg Case Rep 2018;4(1):124.

7. Yokode M, Hanada K, Shimizu A, et al. Intracholecystic papillary neoplasm of the gallbladder protruding into the common bile duct: A case report. Mol Clin Oncol 2019;11(5):488–92.

8. Kiruthiga KG, Kodiatte TA, Burad D, et al. Intracholecystic papillary-tubular neoplasms of the gallbladder - A clinicopathological study of 36 cases. Ann Diagn Pathol 2019;40:88–93.

9. Saei Hamedani F, Garcia-Buitrago M. Pyloric gland adenoma of gallbladder: a review of diagnosis and management. Adv Med 2018;2018:7539694.

10. Saei Hamedani F, Garcia-Buitrago M. Intracholecystic papillary-tubular neoplasms (ICPN) of the gallbladder: a short review of literature. Appl Immunohistochem Mol Morphol 2020;28(1):57–61.

11. Hazarika P, Sharma MK. Intracholecystic papillary-tubular neoplasm of gallbladder: a 5-year retrospective pathological study. Indian J Pathol Microbiol 2018;61(4):516–9.

12. Taskin OC, Akkas G, Memis B, et al. Sarcomatoid carcinomas of the gallbladder: clinicopathologic characteristics. Virchows Arch 2019;475(1):59–66.

13. Roa JC, Tapia O, Cakir A, et al. Squamous cell and adenosquamous carcinomas of the gallbladder: clinicopathological analysis of 34 cases identified in 606 carcinomas. Mod Pathol 2011;24(8):1069–78.

14. de Bitter TJJ, Kroeze LI, de Reuver PR, et al. Unraveling neuroendocrine gallbladder cancer: comprehensive clinicopathologic and molecular characterization. JCO Precis Oncol 2021;5.

15. Yang C, Chen J, Yu Z, et al. Mining of RNA methylation-related genes and elucidation of their molecular biology in gallbladder carcinoma. Front Oncol 2021;11:621806.

16. Iwasaki T, Otsuka Y, Miyata Y, et al. Intracholecystic papillary neoplasm arising in a patient with pancreaticobiliary maljunction: a case report. World J Surg Oncol 2020;18(1):292.

17. Sciarra A, Missiaglia E, Trimech M, et al. Gallbladder mixed neuroendocrine-non-neuroendocrine neoplasm (MiNEN) arising in intracholecystic papillary neoplasm: clinicopathologic and molecular analysis of a case and review of the literature. Endocr Pathol 2020;31(1):84–93.

18. Jones MW, Deppen JG. Gallbladder Polyp. In: StatPearls. Treasure Island (FL): StatPearls Publishing Copyright © 2021, StatPearls Publishing LLC; 2021.

19. Singh A, Singh G, Kaur K, et al. Histopathological changes in gallbladder mucosa associated with cholelithiasis: a prospective study. Niger J Surg 2019;25(1):21–5.

20. Nakanuma Y, Sugino T, Okamura Y, et al. Characterization of high-grade biliary intraepithelial neoplasm of the gallbladder in comparison with intracholecystic papillary neoplasm. Hum Pathol 2021;116:22–30.

21. Xu A, Zhang Y, Hu H, et al. Gallbladder polypoid-lesions: what are they and how should they be treated? a single-center experience based on 1446 cholecystectomy patients. J Gastrointest Surg 2017;21(11):1804–12.

22. Nakanuma Y, Jang KT, Fukushima N, et al. A statement by the Japan-Korea expert pathologists for future clinicopathological and molecular analyses toward consensus building of intraductal papillary neoplasm of the bile duct through several opinions at the present stage. J Hepatobiliary Pancreat Sci 2018;25(3):181–7.

Moving?

Make sure your subscription moves with you!

To notify us of your new address, find your **Clinics Account Number** (located on your mailing label above your name), and contact customer service at:

Email: journalscustomerservice-usa@elsevier.com

800-654-2452 (subscribers in the U.S. & Canada)
314-447-8871 (subscribers outside of the U.S. & Canada)

Fax number: 314-447-8029

Elsevier Health Sciences Division
Subscription Customer Service
3251 Riverport Lane
Maryland Heights, MO 63043

*To ensure uninterrupted delivery of your subscription, please notify us at least 4 weeks in advance of move.

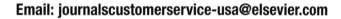
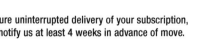
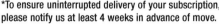

Printed and bound by CPI Group (UK) Ltd, Croydon, CR0 4YY

03/10/2024

01040365-0012